DAILEY'S
NOTES
ON
BLOOD

Third Edition

John F. Dailey

Published by
Medical Consulting Group
Arlington, MA   U.S.A.

Layout by
Desktop Support Consultants
Ipswich, MA

Artwork: Jordan P. Dailey
           Sue Lee
Logo: Susan Keller
Cover Design: Sue Lee

Note: Although the author and publisher have exhaustively researched all sources to ensure the accuracy and completeness of the information contained in this book, we assume no responsibility for errors, inaccuracies, omissions, or any inconsistency herein. Any slights of people or organizations is unintentional. None of the ideas, procedures, or suggestions are intended as substitutes for customary consulting with your physician. All matters regarding your health require medical supervision.

Library of Congress Cataloging-in-Publication Data
Dailey, John F.
Dailey's Notes on Blood
1. Hematology (Science and Health) 2. Immunology (Science and Health)
 ibrary of Congress Card Number: 93-214-993
 ?N: 0-9631819-4-7

 1 in the United States of America
 ?   10 9 8 7 6 5 4 3 2

CONTENTS
Preface
About the Author

CHAPTERS

1   The Concept of Blood   1
   • The Origin of Blood • Bone Marrow • Types of Blood Cells
   • Stem Cells • Growth Factors

2   The Circulatory System   8
   • The Lymphatic System • The Peripheral Circulation
   • The Cardiopulmonary System

3   The Immune System   17
   • Antigens • Antibodies • Humoral and
   Cell-Mediated Responses • The Complement System

4   The ABO and Rh Blood Grouping Systems   25
   • The Rh Antigen

5   Red Blood Cells   31
   • The Function of Hemoglobin
   • The Role of 2, 3-Diphosphoglycerate
   • The Shape of Red Cells • The Number of Red Cells
   • The Role of Erythropoietin • The Hematocrit
   • Red Cell Hemolysis

6   White Blood Cells   41
   • The Number of White Blood Cells • Granulocytes
   • Monocytes/Macrophages • Lymphocytes

7   Plasma   48
   • The Electrolytes and Glucose in Plasma

8   Platelets   53

9   Hemostasis   55
   • Vascular Spasm • Platelet Function in Coagulation
   • Prostaglandins that Regulate ADP Release in Platelet Aggregation
   • Platelet Membrane Phospholipid

10   **The Coagulation Cascade**   61
• The CoagulationPathways • Current Theory of In
Vivo Coagulation • Vitamin K and Coumadin™
• Clot Lysis • Fibrin Split Products

11   **Coagulation System Disorders**   71
• Loss of Vascular Integrity • Coagulation Factor Disorders
• Disseminated Intravascular Coagulation

12   **Platelet Disorders**   76
• Platelet Quality • Platelet Quantity

13   **Blood Transfusion**   79
• Blood Donation • The Citrate Anticoagulants/Preservatives:
CPD, CP2D, and CPDA-1 • Additive Systems • Blood Banking
• Defects in Banked Blood • Blood Grouping and Cross Matching
• Filtering of Blood • Blood Administration

14   **Transfusion Reactions**   90

15   **Transfusion and Disease Transmission**   97
• Hepatitis • HIV • AIDS • Other Transfusion-Transmissible
Diseases

16   **Component Therapy**   104
• Whole Blood in Therapy • Apheresis • Packed Red Cells
• Leukocyte-Poor Red Blood Cells • White Blood Cells • Platelets
• Plasma Components • Albumin and Plasma Protein Fraction
• Immune Serum Globulin • Recombinant Growth Factors

17   **Synthetic Volume Expanders**   118
• Crystalloids • Normal Saline • Lactated Ringer's
• Dextrose • Colloids

18   **The Uses of Autologous Blood**   121
• Predonation • Hemodilution • Intraoperative Blood Salvage
• Postoperative Wound Drainage

Answers to Questions   129
Glossary   145
Appendix   159
• Symbols and Measurements • Normal Blood Values
• Blood Clotting Times • Blood Tests to Evaluate Coagulation
Bibliography   163
Index   165

PREFACE

A thorough understanding of human physiology can only be achieved with a knowledge of blood. In today's world, with the rise of communicable diseases such as AIDS and the resulting need to intensify the testing and screening of blood, the subject of hematology has become critically important. Blood is one of the most fascinating topics in medicine – and one of the most complex. Standard hematology texts require a strong background in the natural sciences and, therefore, the capability for many to acquire an understanding of blood is limited. Author John Dailey recognized that a less technical approach was feasible, practical, and timely. *Dailey's Notes on Blood* provides the reader with a basic working knowledge of blood and its elements and their functions in an easy-to-understand presentation. A knowledge of biology and chemistry is not necessary to use this book as a hematological primer, review, or permanent reference. It is a resource for both the professional and the layperson.

ABOUT MEDICAL CONSULTING GROUP

Medical Consulting Group produces medical publications, provides consulting services, and designs technical training programs for sales personnel and allied health professionals.

The author has two decades of practical experience in surgery and industry including multiple-trauma treatment and operation of the heart bypass pump and other surgical equipment while working with surgeons at a number of New England-area hospitals. Dailey worked in industry for medical equipment manufacturers training physicians and allied health personnel on the use of autologous blood recovery systems in the surgical setting. He also conducted clinical trials on new products; for example, one that collects and processes wound drainage blood and another that is used in the treatment of ischemic heart disease.

Dailey has a B.A. in Biology, St. Francis College, has done graduate studies in biochemistry and physiology at the University of Rhode Island and Brandeis University, and has specialized training in Cardiovascular Perfusion at Northeastern University.

INSTRUCTOR'S OVERHEADS

A boxed set of transparencies is available from the publisher. It includes all figures from the book, a reproduction master for each overhead, and a figure table of contents. Additional figures included are the Circulatory System (anatomical), the Formed Elements, and Blood Clot.

Medical Consulting Group
P.O. Box 1558
Arlington, MA 02174 U.S.A.
1-800-851-8518
617-646-6466
fax: 617-646-4666
mcg@mcgbooks.com

1 The Concept of Blood

A thorough understanding of human physiology can only be achieved with a knowledge of blood. The tissue blood provides an amazingly wide array of life-supporting functions in the human body: (1) it delivers oxygen, hormones, nutrients, and minerals to body cells and picks up cellular waste products; (2) it prevents blood loss by healing wounds; and (3) acts as the primary carrier of immunity. Vital organs not only depend on blood for health, but most are involved in the continuous processing of blood. For example, the heart pumps enormous amounts of blood throughout the body, the kidneys filter out impurities, the liver produces most of the proteins found in blood, and the lungs function in the exchange of oxygen and carbon dioxide between blood and tissues and the external environment.

Hematology is the study of blood and blood-forming tissues. It includes blood's function, diseases, use in surgery and trauma, and role in conditions such as anemia and hemophilia. Hematology is primarily concerned with the formed elements of blood: erythrocytes (red blood cells), leukocytes (white blood cells), and thrombocytes (platelets), all of which are suspended in the liquid medium of blood: plasma. Blood cells may be referred to as formed elements.

hematology

erythrocytes
leukocytes
thrombocytes
plasma
formed elements

Blood is a transportation system, with the vessels of the circulatory system (arteries, veins, and capillaries) functioning as roadways. As blood circulates throughout the body it transports oxygen from the lungs to all body cells for use in cellular reactions. Digestive products absorbed from the intestine are distributed to the cells by the blood. Waste products of cellular metabolism (carbon dioxide and other metabolites) are removed by the blood and delivered to organs such as the lungs, kidneys, and skin for excretion.

The volume of blood present in the circulatory system is referred to as the total blood volume. The average adult

total blood volume   **1**

plasma

has 4 to 6 liters (1 liter = 1000 mL or about 1.06 qts) of blood. Cellular elements make up about 45% of the blood volume and plasma about 55%. Plasma is a viscous fluid that is 90% water and 10% solid matter, the latter consisting of proteins, such as clotting proteins and immunoglobulins, carbohydrates, salts, vitamins, and other substances.

whole blood

Whole blood refers to all of blood's cellular components *and* plasma.

The Origin of Blood

hematopoiesis
bone marrow
stem cell

Hematopoiesis refers to the production of blood cells in the bone marrow. All blood cells develop from a primitive cell called a stem cell that resides in the bone marrow. Blood cell production is an ongoing process in which blood cells are constantly regenerated. Approximately 1 trillion blood cells are produced each day. The production of blood cells is stimulated by different conditions. Low

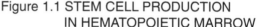

Figure 1.1 STEM CELL PRODUCTION
IN HEMATOPOIETIC MARROW

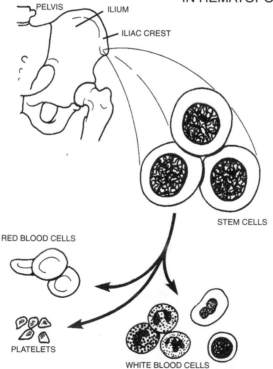

oxygen in the tissues stimulates red cell production. Infection causes an increase in white cell production, and platelet production follows blood loss.

Blood cell development occurs in different sites at various stages of human development. In the yolk sac, a membranous sac that develops in the early embryo, stem cells form clusters of cells called blood islands by the third week of fetal growth. These blood islands are the precursors of blood cells and also the vascular system (blood vessels). By the third month of fetal growth, blood cell production moves from the blood islands to the liver. Thereafter during this month, it takes place in the spleen and thymus. Bone marrow produces all blood cells by the fourth month and continues to do so throughout life. At birth, almost all bones of the body produce blood cells. By adolescence only the flat bones – the skull, sternum, vertebrae, ribs, and pelvis – are involved in blood cell development. In adults the ribs, sternum, vertebrae, and pelvis produce blood cells.

blood islands

Bone Marrow

Bone marrow is a highly complex tissue located in the center of bones. There are two types of marrow: red and yellow. Marrow is made up of a spongy, fibrous matrix called stroma. Hematopoietic (red) marrow consists of 75% water and 25% solid matter, the latter including proteins, carbohydrates, salts, and minerals. Stem cell

stroma
hematopoietic marrow

Figure 1.2 SITES OF BLOOD CELL DEVELOPMENT

 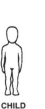 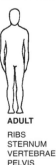

FETUS
YOLK SAC
LIVER
SPLEEN
THYMUS
BONE MARROW

CHILD
SKULL
STERNUM
VERTEBRAE
RIBS, PELVIS
LONG BONES

ADULT
RIBS
STERNUM
VERTEBRAE
PELVIS

Figure 1.3 STEM CELL DIFFERENTIATION

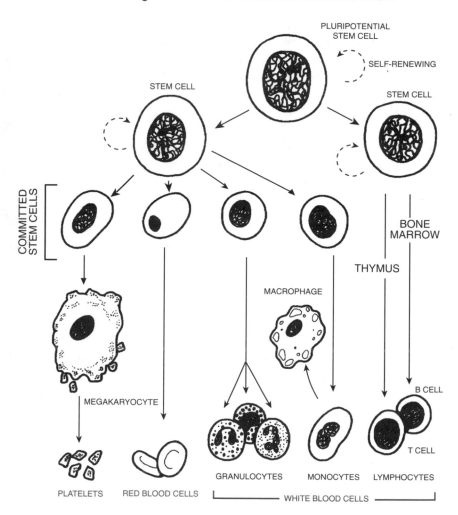

growth and maturation take place within the hematopoietic marrow, which appears as a gelatinous mass within the stroma. Hematopoietic marrow is made up of various cells: fibroblasts, stem cells, endothelial cells, macrophages, and fat cells. Yellow marrow is not involved with hematopoiesis and is 96% fat.

yellow marrow

Blood cell development that occurs in bone marrow is called intramedullary hematopoiesis. When it occurs outside bone marrow, in sites such as the yolk sac, liver, spleen, and thymus, it is called extramedullary hematopoiesis. Unless the bone marrow is diseased or destroyed, extramedullary hematopoiesis does not occur in the adult. Hematopoietic marrow can be destroyed by bone marrow tumors, disease, chemotherapy, radiation, and other causes. Diseased or defective marrow may need to be replaced with healthy marrow from another individual by bone marrow transplant.

intramedullary
hematopoiesis

extramedullary
hematopoiesis

Types of Blood Cells

Each kind of blood cell – red, white, and platelet – has its own function. The white blood cells are part of the immune system, which provides protection against microorganisms and foreign matter. The red blood cells transport oxygen from the lungs to the cells. Platelets are essential in preventing blood loss through platelet plug formation at the site of vascular injury. Once a platelet plug forms, a fibrin clot then forms and stabilizes the plug.

white blood cells
immune system
red blood cells
oxygen
platelets
platelet plug

Blood cells differ structurally from each other, and each has a characteristic life span. In healthy individuals the number of cells in the blood at any time is constant because production and destruction of cells are relatively balanced.

Just as human beings go through the various stages of the life cycle – from birth to death – so do blood cells. For blood cells to carry out their intended function, they must be fully mature. In a healthy person, only mature blood cells are found in the circulation, but in persons with disease states, immature and abnormal cells may be present.

Stem Cells

Fully differentiated, mature blood cells develop from a finite number of stem (progenitor) cells found within the hematopoietic marrow. Stem cells have two functions: (1) the generation of more stem cells, called self-renewal, and (2) the generation of committed blood cells: the red cells, white cells, and platelets. A stem cell is referred to as an undifferentiated cell and the committed, mature blood cell as differentiated. Differentiation is the process of cellular maturation.

committed blood cells

differentiation

pluripotential stem cell

The precursor of all blood cells is the pluripotential stem cell. Most blood cells mature in the hematopoietic marrow, but others mature elsewhere in the body.

Growth Factors

Growth factors are naturally occurring proteins produced by different cells, such as macrophages, activated T lymphocytes, endothelial cells, kidney cells, and fibroblasts. They regulate the growth and differentiation of stem cells into blood cells. When a growth factor binds to a specific protein receptor (binding site) on the stem cell membrane, the stem cell undergoes the change that leads to the process of cellular differentiation.

receptor

stem cell

GM-CSF

G-CSF

EPO

Some examples of growth factors are granulocyte-macrophage colony-stimulating factor (GM-CSF), granulocyte colony-stimulating factor (G-CSF), and erythropoietin (EPO). Advances in molecular biology have enabled researchers to produce growth factors in the laboratory for therapeutic use. Some growth factors have been sanctioned by the Food and Drug Administration (FDA) for use; others are in clinical trials.

Growth factors have a number of therapeutic applications including treatment for patients receiving a bone marrow transplant. They are also used to hasten the recovery of white cells following high-dose chemotherapy. (See Chapter 16.)

Questions

The Concept of Blood

1. Describe two functions of blood essential to human physiology.

2. What are the formed elements of blood? The liquid medium in which they are suspended?

3. Explain why blood is like a transportation system.

4. How many liters of blood does an average adult have?

5. Describe plasma and its components.

6. What does the term hematopoiesis mean and where does it occur in the adult?

7. What condition stimulates the production of red blood cells? White cells? Platelets?

8. Name the two types of bone marrow. Which is involved in blood cell production?

9. Describe the functions of each of the formed elements of blood.

10. What are the two functions of stem cells?

11. What role does the pluripotential stem cell have in blood cell development?

12. Explain the relationship of stem cells and growth factors.

The circulatory system is a closed loop system of the body: blood leaves and returns to the heart. Vessels of the circulatory system carry blood delivering nutrients and oxygen to organs and tissue. Other terms for the circulatory system are the vascular space and vascular system.

vascular space

Fluid continually moves between the circulatory system and tissues. It consists of nutrients, hormones, metabolites (waste products of metabolism), and electrolytes that maintain equilibrium between the blood and tissues of the body. Fluid and plasma components that leave the vascular system enter the interstitial space where they become available to the tissue cells. Interstitial space refers to the space surrounding the cells outside the vascular system. Blood and fluid within the vascular system, or space, is said to be intravascular, and when outside the vascular system, extravascular.

interstititial space
vascular system

intravascular
extravascular

The channels of the vascular system are the arteries, arterioles, capillaries, venules, veins, and indirectly the lymphatic system (see p. 10). The vascular channels are lined with a smooth layer of endothelial cells called the endothelium. Arteries are thick-walled muscular vessels that carry blood away from the heart. Veins are thinner walled, contain less musculature than arteries, and return blood to the heart.

endothelium
arteries
veins

The major artery of the body is the aorta (Ao). It leaves the heart carrying blood for delivery to the cells. The aorta has many arteries branching from it and as these vessels approach organs and tissues they become progressively smaller and are referred to as arterioles. Once inside organs and tissues, arterioles become capillaries, the smallest vessels of the vascular system. Capillaries form a mass of vessels called the capillary network, or capillary bed.

aorta

arterioles

capillary network
capillary bed

Capillaries are the smallest vessels of the vascular system and abound in every organ and tissue of the body. They are

capillaries

Figure 2.1 CIRCULATORY SYSTEM

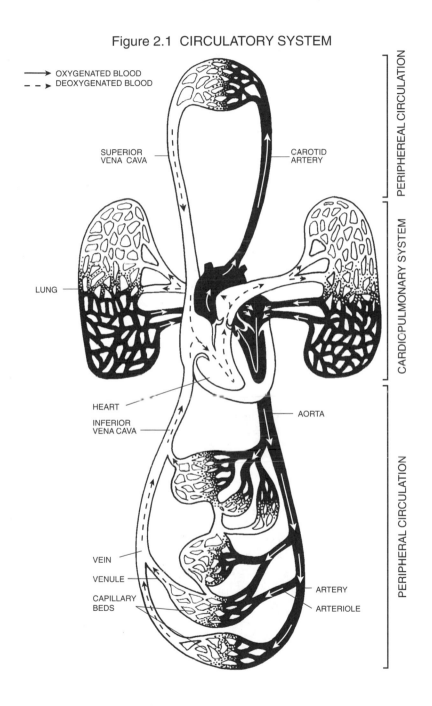

→ OXYGENATED BLOOD
- - → DEOXYGENATED BLOOD

SUPERIOR VENA CAVA

CAROTID ARTERY

LUNG

HEART

INFERIOR VENA CAVA

AORTA

VEIN

VENULE

CAPILLARY BEDS

ARTERY

ARTERIOLE

PERIPHEREAL CIRCULATION

CARDIOPULMONARY SYSTEM

PERIPHERAL CIRCULATION

one cell layer thick, which allows substances to pass easily through them. Capillaries are 1 millimeter (mm) long and 7-9 microns (μ) in diameter. Blood and fluid enter the *arteriolar end* capillary at the arteriolar end of the capillary and exit by the *venule end* venule end.

It is at the capillary level that the exchange of nutrients, gases, hormones, waste products, and other substances takes place between blood and tissues. Pores in the endothelial lining of capillaries expand to allow substances to pass between the blood and tissues by the processes of *filtration* filtration, osmosis, and diffusion. Large, molecular-weight *osmosis* substances that leave the vascular system and pass through *diffusion* the capillary pores often are unable to return to the capillary. They are picked up and returned to the circulation by *lymphatic channels* a network of vessels called lymphatic channels. Fluid that does not leave the capillary is returned through the venules to the veins and on to the heart.

The Lymphatic System

The lymphatic system is a network of capillarylike vessels, ducts, nodes, and organs that help maintain the fluid environment of the body. Like the blood-vascular system, the lymphatic system is made up of a system of channels. It

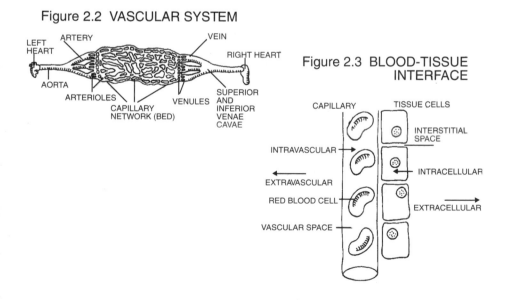

Figure 2.2 VASCULAR SYSTEM

Figure 2.3 BLOOD-TISSUE INTERFACE

Figure 2.4 LYMPHATIC SYSTEM

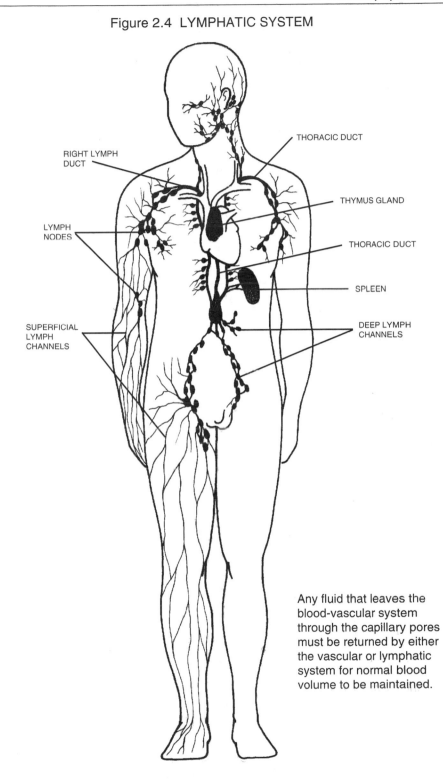

RIGHT LYMPH DUCT

LYMPH NODES

SUPERFICIAL LYMPH CHANNELS

THORACIC DUCT

THYMUS GLAND

THORACIC DUCT

SPLEEN

DEEP LYMPH CHANNELS

Any fluid that leaves the blood-vascular system through the capillary pores must be returned by either the vascular or lymphatic system for normal blood volume to be maintained.

does the following: (1) picks up fluids and large complex substances that have left the circulatory system and entered the tissues and (2) returns them to the vascular system by way of the thoracic and right lymphatic ducts.

lymph

Fluid in the lymphatic channels is called lymph.

The lymphatic system does not form a closed loop system like the vascular system. Lymphatic vessels begin as tiny, unconnected capillarylike structures in tissues. These structures merge to form progressively larger vessels that are

lymph nodes

interrupted at various sites by lymph nodes, which are small filtering stations of particulate matter and antigen.

Lymphatic vessels drain into two large lymph vessels, the

thoracic duct

right lymphatic duct

thoracic duct on the left side of the body and the right lymphatic duct on the right side. These two vessels empty into veins in the upper chest and return fluid to the vascular system.

Any fluid that leaves the vascular system through the capillary must ultimately be returned to the capillary by osmosis, filtration, and diffusion or picked up by the

blood volume

lymphatic system. Blood volume is thus maintained.

Fluid leaves the vascular system due to pressure differences between the blood and tissues and in the process delivers nutrients to the cells. Blood pressure filters fluid from the arteriolar end of the capillary into the interstitial space.

plasma proteins

osmotic pressure

Plasma proteins remain in the capillaries where they exert osmotic pressure that pulls this fluid back into the circulation at the venule end of the capillary. If fluid remains in the interstitial space, the individual develops a swollen appearance, a condition called edema. Furthermore, blood volume is depleted from the circulation. Plasma proteins are essential in helping to maintain blood volume.

Fluids of the body require constant circulation, and the pump that maintains circulation is the heart. The heart propels fluids through the blood-vascular system.

The Peripheral Circulation

The vascular system includes the peripheral and cardio-pulmonary systems. The peripheral circulation refers to the arteries, arterioles, venules, and veins that are outside the chest. It is not part of the cardiopulmonary circulation, which refers to the blood vessels of the heart and lungs.

The circulatory system can be thought of as one large continuous loop: arteries take blood away from the heart and veins return blood to the heart. Arteries branch from the aorta and become smaller to form arterioles, which branch further to form capillaries. At the distal (farthest) end of the capillaries, the venules form. They are the smallest veins. As venules return blood to the heart, they become progressively larger to form veins. The veins return blood to the heart through the two major veins of the body, the superior vena cava and the inferior vena cava. The superior vena cava receives venous blood from the head and upper part of the body, whereas the inferior vena cava receives venous blood from the lower part of the body. These two vessels enter the right atrium of the heart.

arteries
arterioles
capillaries

venules
veins

superior vena cava
inferior vena cava

Figure 2.5 HEART

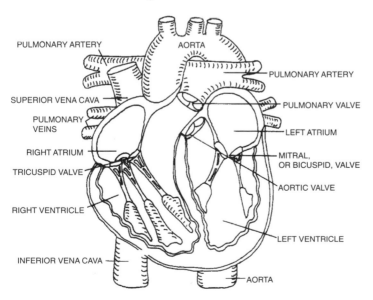

The Cardiopulmonary System

The cardiopulmonary system refers to the heart and lungs as they function together. The heart pumps blood throughout the body and to the lungs where blood receives oxygen. Blood that returns from the organs and tissues is low in oxygen and high in carbon dioxide. Deoxygenated blood passes through the inferior and superior venae cavae to the

right atrium
right ventricle
tricuspid valve
pulmonary valve
and artery

right atrium (RA) of the heart. Blood in the right atrium is pumped to the right ventricle (RV) through the tricuspid valve. Blood is then pumped from the right ventricle out through the pulmonary valve to the pulmonary artery, which divides and goes to each lung.

lungs

The lungs are large spongy organs filled with capillaries and alveoli. The microvasculature (capillary network) of the lungs is very large. In fact, if this system were removed and spread out it would be the size of a tennis court. The capillaries of the lungs form a close network with the

alveoli
alveolar-capillary
network

oxygen
carbon dioxide

alveoli, which are tiny air sacs within the lungs filled with oxygen. It is in the alveolar-capillary network that oxygen and carbon dioxide are exchanged between blood and the environment. Carbon dioxide is the waste product of cellular metabolism. Once the exchange of gases has taken place, oxygenated blood is returned from the lungs by the

left atrium
left ventricle
mitral valve
aortic valve

aorta

pulmonary veins to the left atrium (LA) of the heart. Blood in the left atrium is pumped into the left ventricle (LV) through the mitral (bicuspid) valve. The oxygen-rich blood is ejected from the left ventricle through the aortic valve to the aorta. From there, blood is distributed throughout the body by arteries, arterioles, and capillaries.

Figure 2.6 CARDIOPULMONARY SYSTEM

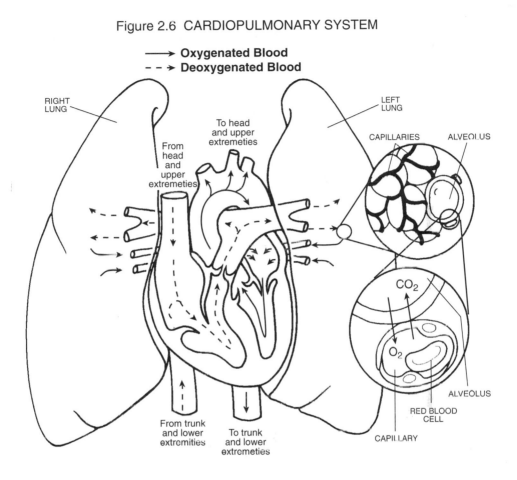

Questions

The Circulatory System

1. Explain the relationship between blood and the circulatory system.

2. What happens to fluid in the interstitial space?

3. Describe the path that blood follows when it leaves the heart and goes to the tissues and organs.

4. What important physiological function takes place at the capillary level?

5. What is the major function of the lymphatic system?

6. Describe the role of plasma proteins in maintaining blood volume.

7. Define the peripheral circulation. The cardiopulmonary system.

8. What is the lining of the vascular system called?

9. What is deoxygenated blood?

10. Describe the pathway of dexoygenated blood in the cardiopulmonary system.

11. What two gases are exchanged in the alveolar capillary network of the lungs?

12. Describe the pathway of oxygenated blood in the cardiopulmonary system.

3 | The Immune System

During the last few decades, important discoveries have been made about the immune system and how it functions. A knowledge of the immune system is incomplete without an understanding of hematology and the roles of the white blood cells (leukocytes).

leukocytes

The immune system protects the body from microorganisms and foreign substances by attacking them and rendering them harmless. This reaction to invaders is the immune response and involves complement proteins, antibodies, and white blood cells: granulocytes, macrophages, and lymphocytes. A complicated task faces the specialized organs, tissues, and white blood cells that make up the immune system: to recognize and destroy harmful invaders without causing damage to the body's own tissue.

immune response
antibodies
complement proteins
granulocytes
macrophages
lymphocytes

The immune system is unlike any of the body's other systems. It is not a system of channels like the circulatory system or an electrical network like the nervous system. The various components of the immune system move freely throughout the body penetrating both fluids and tissues.

A useful way to understand the immune system is to think of it as a highly trained and disciplined military unit. It consists of training and support groups, specialized units, and a highly skilled communications network. Surveillance units are constantly on the lookout for foreign invaders and provide the first line of defense for the body. When encountering foreign organisms they send signals that activate unit members to mount the necessary defense to prevent the invaders from reaching their target.

Antigens

Antigens (Ags) are any group of microorganisms or foreign matter, other people's cells, tumor cells, and virally infected cells that enter the body and initiate the immune

microorganisms
foreign matter
immune response **17**

response. The body recognizes antigens as not part of "self." Microorganisms include bacteria, viruses, and some parasites. Technically, antigens are molecules, or portions thereof, of the proteins, carbohydrates, and lipids on the surface of the invaders. Antigens are introduced into the body by various routes; for example, through the skin, mouth, and blood.

Antibodies

An antibody (Ab) is a chemically complex protein molecule produced by B cells/plasma cells in response to an antigen. When a B cell recognizes an antigen it matures into a plasma cell, which produces a specific corresponding antibody that coats (opsonises) the antigen. An opsonin is a molecule, such as antibody or complement protein, that adheres to antigen. Opsonization makes antigen more palatable to phagocytic cells. Once an antigen-antibody complex is formed, antigen can be destroyed by phagocytic white blood cells that have become activated in seeking out and engulfing the complex.

B cells/plasma cells

opsonization
antigen-antibody
complex

Antibodies, also called immunoglobulins, are divided into five classes and released on exposure to antigen. On reexposure to the same antigen, the corresponding antibody is produced in greater amounts.

IgM

I. IgM (immunoglobulin M) is the first antibody produced on exposure to an antigen. It is a large, chemically complex molecule, which because of its size is restricted to remain within the vasculature; it cannot escape into the tissues. Its main function is to stimulate the complement system. (See p. 21.)

IgD

II. Little is known about the IgD antibody. Researchers believe it assists the maturation of the B cell into a plasma cell. Very low concentrations are found in the plasma. IgD probably has very little protective function.

IgE

III. The antibody IgE is produced in excess in people with allergies and parasitic infections. Most of the white blood cells that rush to the defense of attacked tissue do so through the bloodstream. IgE is specifically designed to stimulate basophils and mast cells to release histamine, the chemical that causes pores in the capillary wall to dilate and allow white cells to enter the tissue. As soon as this occurs, IgE has performed its function.

IV. IgG is the immunoglobulin most important to humans. It is produced in greatest amounts on second exposure to antigen. This immunoglobulin is divided into four subgroups, each of which has a specific purpose. IgG_1 protects the body from bacteria, except those encased in a saccharide (sugar) coat; for example, meningococcus, pneumococcus, and gonococcus. IgG_2, attacks and destroys these organisms. IgG_3 binds complement proteins, a process that enhances the destruction of antigen by phagocytosis. IgG_4 is similar to IgE that it produces potent vasodilators, which are substances that cause vessel pores to open. IgG_4 primarily provides protection for the bronchioles (airways) of the respiratory tract (lungs).

IgG

V. IgA, the fifth class of antibodies, protects mucous membranes that line mouth, bladder, gut, nose, and vagina and forms a protective barrier for these areas. IgA simply binds the antigen and immobilizes it so that the antigen-antibody complex can be removed with mucin, a viscous fluid produced by mucous membranes.

IgA

Humoral and Cell-Mediated Responses

The immune response is divided into two branches: the cell-mediated and humoral. They work together to defeat antigen.

Cell-mediated (T cell) responses occur between antigens and specialized lymphocytes known as T cells. When T cells recognize antigen they direct the appropriate immune cells to respond to antigen and destroy it. T cells are stimulated by certain antigens, such as foreign cells, to become cytoxic and therefore capable of destroying antigen by lysis, which is the disruption by toxins of the cell membrane leading to cell death. (See Lymphocytes, p. 45.)

cell-mediated responses
T cell

cytoxic
lysis

Cell-mediated responses are crucial for combating infections caused by microorganisms that reside and multiply

intracellular attack

within cells. Viruses and some bacteria prefer intracellular attack, which involves attacking the cell from inside rather than outside the cell membrane. It is within the cell that viruses replicate and do most of their damage. Cell-mediated responses also destroy tumor (cancer) and allogeneic (some one else's) cells.

humoral responses
B cells/plasma cells
antibody

macrophage

Humoral (antibody) responses are carried out by B cells/plasma cells through the production and circulation of antibody in response to an antigen. When antibody complexes with antigen the antigen becomes more palatable to the macrophage, a large white blood cell. The antigen is then destroyed by phagocytosis when macrophages and neutrophils engulf it. In some instances, antibody production is increased when B cells are stimulated by T cells. Antibody is effective against antigen outside the cell but powerless once antigen enters the cell.

phagocytosis

Phagocytosis is the process by which white blood cells, mainly macrophages and neutrophils, engulf foreign ma-

Figure 3.1 IMMUNE RESPONSE

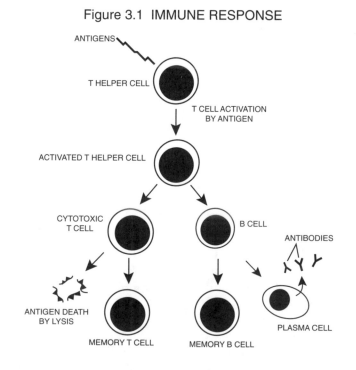

terial and render it harmless through the action of enzymes located in their cytoplasm. Phagocytosis occurs when macrophages and neutrophils are stimulated by molecules released by T lymphocytes. The phagocytic process can follow both the humoral and cell-mediated responses.

macrophages
neutrophils

The Complement System

The complement system is a group of 18 to 20 naturally occurring soluble proteins dissolved in the blood plasma that provide immune protection. They circulate in the inactive form throughout the body becoming activated on exposure to antigen and in the inflammatory response to tissue injury. Complement becomes activated in the presence of antigen and attacks antigen as soon as antigen enters the body.

complement proteins

antigen

The function of the complement system is to generate activated complement proteins that lead to antigen destruction and the repair of injured tissue. Complement provides a first-line defense against antigen and is independent of other immune system components – such as white blood cells and antibodies. Complement and antibodies differ in that antibodies need time to be produced in sufficient amounts to defeat antigen. Also, antibodies increase in numbers on exposure to the antigen whereas complement proteins do not.

There are instances when complement proteins are activated in the absence of activating antigen; for example, during open heart surgery, hemodialysis, and when autologous blood is collected during or after surgery. For reasons not really clear, foreign surfaces have the capability of stimulating the complement system. The tubing and equipment used in certain procedures activates complement proteins, which can destroy normal healthy cells.

foreign surfaces

A manifestation of inappropriate complement system activation is hemolysis, the destruction of red blood cell membranes. Hemolysis is a potentially lethal situation for the individual. If it becomes widespread and a large number of red cells is destroyed, very few red cells are left to transport oxygen to the tissues. Remnants of the hemo-

hemolysis

lyzed red cells initiate the coagulation cascade. Clots then form and block the microvasculature of the lungs and kidneys.

Certain genetic disorders affect the production of complement proteins. The disorders can cause a total deficiency of complement proteins or a reduction in their number. Both disorders render affected individuals susceptible to constant bacterial infections.

Complement Protein Activation

Complement proteins become activated in a chain reaction sequence that leads to antigen destruction. Once activated, complement molecules split (cleave) other complement proteins that split still other complement proteins. Activated complement proteins are responsible for generating molecules essential to immune activity.

Complement proteins have several functions in antigen destruction. (1) Some complement components increase vascular permeability, which allows white blood cells to move into the area of antigen invasion. (2) Other complement proteins assist phagocytosis by coating (opsonizing) antigen. (3) Other complement components adhere to antigen and rupture the antigen's membrane, a process referred to as lysis (see below).

vascular permeability

phagocytosis

lysis

The Complement Pathways

Evolution has provided two complement pathways within the complement system: the classical and the alternative. The pathways are distinct because each is activated by different antigens. The classical pathway is activated by antigen-antibody complexes and the alternative pathway is activated by certain bacteria, aggregates of some antibodies, and toxins (poisons) produced by bacteria. When the complement system is activated it generates active complement proteins that lead to antigen destruction.

classical pathway

The classical pathway consists of 9 complement proteins. They become activated by antigens, such as microorganisms, allogeneic (someone else's) cells, and tumor (malignant) cells that have been opsonized by either IgM or IgG antibodies. Classical pathway complement proteins adhere to antigen coated with IgM or IgG antibody, thereby enhancing phagocytosis.

The alternative pathway consists of 5 complement proteins. This pathway is activated by bacteria with polysaccharide capsules (outer coverings), aggregates of IgA and IgE antibodies, the cell wall of microorganisms, such as yeast, and potent chemical toxins produced by certain bacteria.

alternative pathway

The membrane attack complex (MAC) forms following the activation of either complement pathway. It consists of 5 complement proteins that conclude the complement system's chain reaction through either pathway. The MAC proteins attach to an antigen's cell membrane and bore (lyse) holes in it, causing the antigen to lose fluid and, therefore, its destruction.

MAC

Figure 3.2 COMPLEMENT SYSTEM

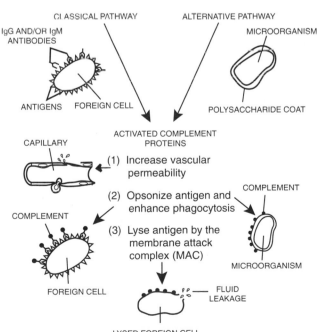

Questions

The Immune System

1.   What is the primary function of the immune system?

2.   Which formed elements are involved in the immune system?

3.   Define antigens.

4.   What is an antibody and what cell produces it?

5.   How is an antigen-antibody complex formed?

6.   What is another term for antibody?

7.   Provide two reasons why IgG is the most important immunoglobulin to humans.

8.   True or false: Antibodies cannot penetrate a cell's membrane.

9.   What are the two branches of the immune response and how does each function in providing immunity?

10.   Why are viruses protected from the effects of antibodies?

11.   What is phagocytosis and when does it occur?

12.   What is complement and how does it interact with antibodies?

13.   Name the complement pathways and explain how each functions.

14.   What is the function of the membrane attack complex?

4 | The ABO and Rh Blood Grouping Systems

Blood groups were discovered at the beginning of the twentieth century by Karl Landsteiner, an Austrian hematologist. Blood groups in the ABO system are determined by the presence of two distinct antigens (complex carbohydrates) found on the surface of the red blood cell membrane. The antigens are inherited from one's parents and designated "A" and "B." Red blood cells with the A antigen on their surface membrane are called group A, those with the B antigen group B, those with both antigens A and B group AB, and those with neither antigen present group O.

A and B antigens
red cell membrane

Landsteiner also discovered two natural antibodies in the blood plasma: anti-A antibody and anti-B antibody. Persons with group A blood have anti-B antibody in their plasma; those with group B blood have the anti-A antibody. The plasma of group AB blood has neither antibody in it, whereas group O blood has both anti-A and anti-B antibodies in the plasma. The anti-A antibody in group B blood agglutinates (clumps) the red blood cells in group A blood. Anti-B antibody in group A agglutinates group B blood cells. Neither antibody agglutinates group O blood cells, because there are no antigens on group O red cell membranes. When the antigens on the red cells of a blood donor agglutinate with the antibodies in the plasma of the recipient, the blood groups are incompatible. The wrong blood group has been administered and the patient experiences a hemolytic transfusion reaction. (See Chapter 14.)

antibodies
blood plasma

agglutination

Medical personnel must be sure of the patient's blood group: it can be fatal if the wrong blood group is administered. When allogeneic (someone else's) blood is transfused its group must be compatible with the patient's. A group A patient must receive group A or O packed cells and a group B patient group B or O packed cells. A group AB patient can receive the following groups: A, B, AB, or O packed cells. Group O can receive only group O packed cells.

allogeneic blood

Figure 4.1 ABO BLOOD GROUPING COMPATIBILITY

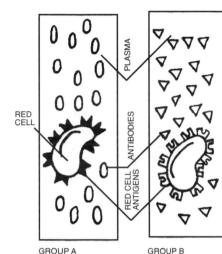

GROUP A
ANTI-B ANTIBODY

GROUP B
ANTI-A ANTIBODY

GROUP AB
NO ANTIBODIES
BOTH ANTIGENS

GROUP O
ANTI-A AND
ANTI-B ANTIBODIES
NO ANTIGENS

CROSS MATCHING

I = Incompatible
C= Compatible

To determine blood compatibility for transfusion purposes, recipient serum (plasma minus fibrinogen) is mixed with the red cells of various donors. If the cells do not clump, a donor's blood can be mixed with the recipient's blood in a transfusion.

RECIPIENT BLOOD GROUP

DONOR BLOOD GROUP (PACKED RED CELLS ONLY)	O	A	B	AB
O	C	C	C	C
A	I	C	I	C
B	I	I	C	C
AB	I	I	I	C

In the early days of blood transfusion, group O blood was considered the "universal donor" because there are no antigens on its red blood cell membrane. Group AB blood was considered the "universal recipient" because there are no antibodies in its plasma. Today, identical blood groups are preferentially used, but group O- red blood cells may be administered in an emergency when a specific group is unavailable.

universal donor

universal recipient

What happens when an individual receives an incompatible blood group? He or she experiences what is known as a hemolytic transfusion reaction in which destruction of the donor red blood cells occurs. The reaction happens when donor and recipient red blood cells are incompatible. The most severe symptoms in such a case may include shock, chills, fever, chest pain, dyspnea (shortness of breath), back pain, and/or abnormal bleeding. Death may also result. For an anesthetized patient, hypotension (low blood pressure) and evidence of disseminated intravascular coagulation (DIC; see p.72) may be the first indications that the wrong blood group has been used. Administration of the wrong blood group is usually due to clerical error.

hemolytic transfusion reaction

The Rh Antigen

There are important red cell antigen groups in addition to ABO. The next most important is the Rh, also called the D antigen. The Rh antigen was originally discovered in the Rhesus monkey, hence "Rh." It may or may not be present on the red cell membrane. A + sign indicates its presence and a - sign the absence of the Rh antigen. The ABO and Rh systems are often designated together. For example, an individual may have A+ blood, A-, and so on.

As with the ABO blood group there is a risk of a reaction to the Rh antigen, especially for the individual who does not have it. The first time an Rh- person receives Rh+ blood there may be few complications due to incompatibility. However, a subsequent transfusion of Rh+ blood is potentially lethal because by then the Rh- recipient has developed antibodies to the Rh+ blood from the previous transfusion and will destroy the newly transfused red cells.

Figure 4.2 Rh- MOTHER WITH Rh+ FETUS

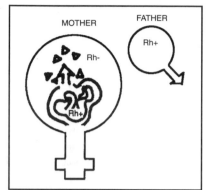

1. FIRST PREGNANCY

- NO HARM TO FETUS
- NO PROBLEMS FOR MOTHER

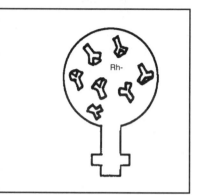

2. BEFORE AND AFTER DELIVERY
   OF FIRST CHILD

- MOTHER HAS DEVELOPED
  ANTIBODIES TO Rh+ ANTIGEN
  OF THE FETUS

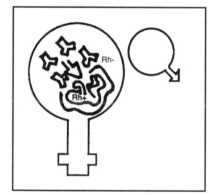

3. SECOND PREGNANCY

- MOTHER'S ANTIBODIES ATTACK
  FETAL BLOOD CELLS
- HDN OCCURS

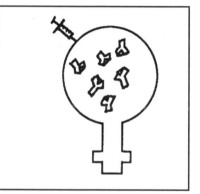

Rh IMMUNE GLOBULIN PREVENTS
MOTHER'S ANTIBODIES FROM FORMING

Rh IMMUNE GLOBULIN CAN BE ADMINISTERED:
- TO AN Rh- MOTHER WITH AN Rh+ FETUS
- ANY TIME THERE IS A MIX OF BLOOD
  BETWEEN MOTHER AND FETUS (e.g.,
  ECTOPIC PREGNANCY,
  MISCARRIAGE, AMNIOCENTESIS)
- TO AN Rh- WOMAN NEEDING Rh+ PLATELETS
- AFTER EACH Rh+ CHILD

The patient has a severe immune reaction and may possibly die. Unlike antibodies in the ABO group, antibodies to Rh are not preformed but develop after exposure to the Rh antigen.

A commonly used example to illustrate the significance of the Rh antigen is an Rh- mother and an Rh+ father who have a baby that is Rh+. In this case, any fetal blood that leaks across the placenta stimulates the mother's immune system to make antibodies against the Rh+ blood of the fetus. The Rh antigen usually poses no threat to the first fetus. In later pregnancies an Rh+ fetus is in jeopardy because the antibodies produced by the mother in the first pregnancy will attack fetal blood and may cause a condition known as hemolytic disease of the newborn (HDN).   HDN

Doctors can now prevent HDN by injecting the mother with Rh immune globulin, which neutralizes antibodies   Rh immune globulin
produced against the Rh antigen. If HDN does occur, an exchange transfusion either in utero or following delivery can prevent fetal death.

Questions

The ABO and Rh Blood Grouping Systems

1. How are blood groups identified in the ABO system?

2. State the blood group identified with the presence of each of the following red cell antigens: a. A and B   b. A antigen   c. B antigen

3. How is group O blood different from other blood groups in the ABO system?

4. What two natural antibodies appear in blood and in what portion are they found?

5. What antibody appears in each of the following blood groups: A, B, O, AB?

6. How do antibodies interact with antigens on the red cell membrane?

7. Explain why neither anti-A nor anti-B antibody agglutinates group O blood cells.

8. What happens when donor blood and recipient blood are incompatible?

9. When is universal group O blood administered?

10. Why does the Rh antigen present the risk of a transfusion reaction following the intitial transfusion?

11. True or false: An Rh+ individual can receive multiple transfusions of Rh- blood. Explain your answer.

12. What treatment can be given to an Rh- mother to neutralize the antibodies produced against the Rh+ antigen of the fetus?

5 | Red Blood Cells

As the red blood cells ready themselves for expulsion from the bone marrow into the circulation, the endothelial lining of the capillary in the bone marrow develops a pore. The red cell squeezes through the pore, whereupon the nucleus is pinched off. The enucleated mature red cells are released from the marrow into the circulation and have a life span of approximately 120 days. Red blood cells are called erythrocytes. They deliver oxygen to the tissues and return carbon dioxide from the tissues to the lungs.

ERYTHROCYTE
(RED BLOOD CELL)

erythrocytes
oxygen
carbon dioxide

Unlike most cells of the body, mature red cells, once in the circulation, do not contain a nucleus. There are three reasons for this. (1) The main function of a red blood cell is the transport of oxygen and carbon dioxide. The presence of a nucleus would decrease the amount of space available to these gases. (2) The nucleus of a cell has a certain mass. Nucleated red cells would add significantly to the weight of the blood and increase the workload of the heart by about 20%. (3) Red cells are fully differentiated and do not require a nucleus to carry out the function of transporting oxygen and carbon dioxide.

The Function of Hemoglobin

The primary function of red blood cells is the transport of oxygen. This process is made possible by a chemically complex protein molecule present in the red cells called hemoglobin (Hgb). During circulation of blood through the lungs, Hgb becomes almost fully saturated with oxygen, making the blood bright red. As red cells perfuse the capillary beds of tissues and organs, oxygen is released from Hgb to the tissues.

transport of oxygen

Hgb

In the red cells of normal adults, Hgb consists of two alpha (α) and two beta (β) chains, with a heme molecule attached to each chain. These chains consist of amino acids, which are the building blocks of proteins. The heme molecule attached to each chain is responsible for the red color of blood. The biosynthesis (production) of Hgb takes place

heme molecule

Figure 5.1 STRUCTURE OF HEMOGLOBIN

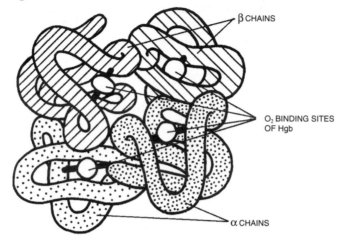

β CHAINS

O₂ BINDING SITES
OF Hgb

α CHAINS

Figure 5.2 ALVEOLAR CAPILLARY NETWORK

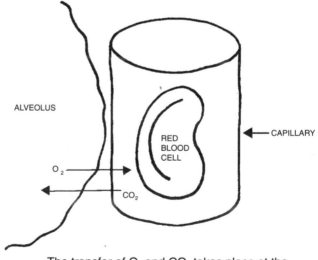

ALVEOLUS

RED
BLOOD
CELL

CAPILLARY

O₂

CO₂

The transfer of O_2 and CO_2 takes place at the
alveolar capillary network of the lung.

in a cellular structure of immature red blood cells known as the mitochondria. When the mature red cell enters the circulation from the bone marrow it loses the mitochondria as well as the nucleus.

The main function of Hgb is the transport of oxygen from the lungs to the tissues, therefore, the concentration of Hgb in a patient is a matter of concern. Almost all body functions depend on the oxygen-transport capability of the blood. When the Hgb concentration is low, tissues may not receive an adequate amount of oxygen, and over time this presents problems. Inadequate oxygen supply to tissues results in poor healing of tissue and can cause complications such as an increased workload on the heart.

An accurate indication of the oxygen carrying capacity of blood can be taken by measuring the concentration of Hgb. The normal Hgb concentrations for males are 13.5 - 18.0 g/dL and for females 12.0 - 16.0 g/dL.

The oxygen that tissues receive depends on three conditions: (1) the amount of blood flow to the tissues, (2) the level of Hgb concentration in the blood, and (3) the affinity of Hgb for oxygen. Patients with an abnormality of one of the factors automatically compensate by adjusting one or both of the other two factors so that optimal tissue perfusion (oxygenation) is maintained. For example,   tissue perfusion

Figure 5.3 OXYGEN-CARBON DIOXIDE TRANSFER

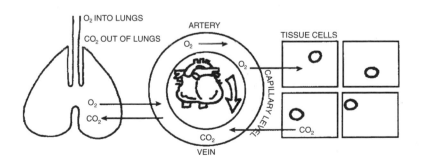

if the Hgb concentration is low, the body compensates by increasing the heart rate, which in turn increases the amount of blood delivered to the tissues.

pH
PCO$_2$
2,3-DPG

The affinity of Hgb for oxygen is regulated by three factors: (1) hydrogen ion concentration, or pH; (2) the partial pressure of carbon dioxide (PCO$_2$); and (3) the chemical 2,3-diphosphoglycerate (2,3-DPG). If one of these three factors is not within its normal limits, Hgb will not release oxygen as readily to the tissues. (See Normal Values in Appendix.)

The Role of 2,3-Diphosphoglycerate

Another important chemical found in red cells is 2,3-diphosphoglycerate (DPG). This molecule is present in the same concentration as Hgb in the blood and is bound to Hgb. The function of 2,3-DPG is to lower Hgb's affinity for oxygen so that Hgb releases oxygen to the tissues more easily. Without 2,3-DPG, Hgb would release little oxygen to the tissues.

stored blood

The discovery of the role of 2,3-DPG in oxygen release to tissues has provided clinical medicine with new insights about stored blood, which has very low levels of 2,3-DPG. When patients receive large volumes of stored blood, the amount of oxygen released to the tissues is minimal and can cause serious problems. Furthermore, transfused cells depleted of 2,3-DPG can regain only half their normal level in a 24-hour period, which may not be rapid enough for a patient already compromised or severely ill. Adding 2,3-DPG to stored blood is of little value because the red cell membrane is impermeable to (will not allow in) this molecule.

It has been shown that 2,3-DPG is an important regulator of Hgb function. The chemical 2,3-DPG also aids Hgb's uptake of oxygen in the lungs.

The Shape of Red Blood Cells

Red blood cells are flexible, biconcave disks with a diameter of 7 μ and a thickness of 2 μ. This shape gives the red cell a maximum surface area and thus facilitates the transfer of gases into and out of the cell. The flexibility of the red cell also enables it easily to undergo the changes in shape necessary for travel through the capillaries of the body. The capillaries are only slightly larger than the red blood cells.

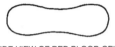

SIDE VIEW OF RED BLOOD CELL

The Number of Red Blood Cells

The number of red blood cells in the average adult is 4.2-6.2 x 10^{12}/L. (The average number of red blood cells is usually 5.5 x 10^{12}/L for males and 4.5 x 10^{12}/L for females.) This number is standard, and any deviation from it suggests a problem. If there are too many red cells in the circulation or a high red cell count exists, the condition is referred to as either erythrocytosis or polycythemia. It is often seen in patients with cyanotic heart disease.

erythrocytosis or polycythemia

A high red cell number may cause circulatory problems; for example, the blood is so thick that it blocks the microvasculature of the lungs and kidneys. A low red cell count is termed anemia and is often seen in patients receiving chemotherapy or radiation therapy for cancer and in end-stage renal disease. Anemia indicates there are not enough red cells in the circulation to transport sufficient amounts of oxygen to the tissues. With anemia, other body systems have to compensate to deliver an adequate amount of oxygen to the tissues. For example, the heart beats faster and breathing becomes more rapid as the lungs take in air.

anemia

Figure 5.4 RELEASE OF ERYTHROPOIETIN

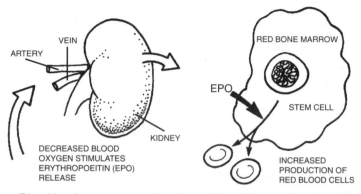

Blood low in oxygen passing through the kidneys stimulates the release of erythropoietin (EPO), which then stimulates stem cells in the bone marrow to develop into red blood cells. An increase in numbers of red blood cells increases the oxygen-carrying capacity of blood.

Figure 5.5 HEMATOCRITS

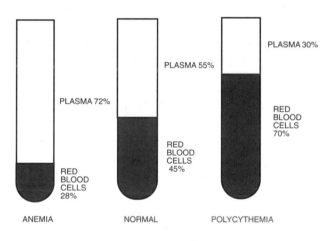

The Role of Erythropoietin

The production of red cells is termed erythropoiesis. It is initiated by erythropoietin, which is a hormone produced and released by the kidneys and circulated in the plasma. When a person's Hgb level is below normal, which can happen for a number of reasons, the tissues do not receive enough oxygen. A low level of oxygen in tissues is called hypoxia. In hypoxia the kidneys are stimulated to increase the production of erythropoietin, whereupon the stem cells in the marrow are activated to produce more red cells.

erythropoiesis
erythropoietin

hypoxia

The Hematocrit

An important factor in red cell physiology is the hematocrit (Hct), which is the percentage of whole blood occupied by the red blood cells. The Hct is considered to be an index of the red cell concentration and thus an indirect measure of the oxygen-carrying capacity of the blood. In the normal adult the Hct is between 0.38-0.54 (38%-54%). This range indicates that 0.38-0.54 of whole blood is made up of red cells. Remember, white cells and platelets make up only 0.01 of the Hct.

Hct

The Hct and Hgb are related: the Hct is approximately three times the value of the Hgb. For example, if a patient's Hgb is 15 g/dL (grams per deciliter), then the Hct should be about 0.45. When the formed elements make up 0.45 of the blood, then the other 0.55 consists of plasma. A unit of stored allogeneic red cells when transfused into the average-sized adult elevates the Hct by about 0.03-0.04. For example, if the Hct is 0.35, a unit of red cells raises it to 0.38.

Red Cell Hemolysis

immune response

sepsis
stress

spleen

plasma-free Hgb

stroma

Hemolysis refers to the destruction of the red cell membrane and is a serious problem. It may be caused by a number of factors: (1) the immune response; for example, when a unit of the wrong blood group is administered or in an autoimmune reaction, (2) sepsis (bacterial or viral infection), and (3) red cell membrane stress caused by high suction pressure from autologous blood recovery devices, the cardiac bypass pump, the hemodialysis machine, and other equipment.

As red blood cells age their membranes become fragile and more easily hemolyzed. Older cells near the end of their life cycle are normally removed by the spleen, which is an organ located in the upper left-hand corner of the abdomen under the ribs. Hemolyzed cells, due to whatever cause, can present problems to patients. When the cell ruptures Hgb is released, causing a condition called plasma-free Hgb. Hgb can no longer transport oxygen, so the blood's ability to oxygenate tissue is decreased. The cell stroma (remnant of the ruptured cell) stimulate clot formation that may block the microvasculature of the lungs and kidneys, causing these organs to fail.

Figure 5.6 RED BLOOD CELL HEMOLYSIS

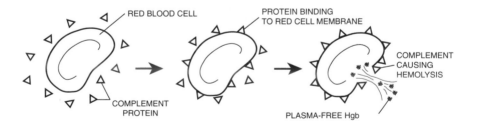

One cause of red cell hemolysis is the oposinization of complement protein on the red cell membrane.

Questions

Red Blood Cells

1. What is the term used for red blood cells?

2. Where are red blood cells formed and what is their approximate life span?

3. Describe the main function of the red blood cell.

4. Give one reason why the red cell contains no nucleus.

5. What is the name of the complex protein molecule present in red blood cells? Its acronym?

6. Describe the role hemoglobin has in getting oxygen to the tissues.

7. Why is blood the color red?

8. Explain why normal patient physiology depends on Hgb.

9. What three factors contribute to the optimal perfusion (oxygenation) of tissues that is vital for health?

10. What three factors regulate the affinity of hemoglobin for oxygen? If one of the factors is not within normal limits, what is the consequence?

11. What role does 2,3,-DPG have in the release of oxygen to the tissues?

12. What serious problem may be posed to a patient who receives many transfusions of stored blood?

13. The shape of a red blood cell is significant. Give one reason why.

14. Polycythemia and anemia are disorders associated with the number of red blood cells in the circulation. Describe the implications of each condition to the patient.

15.   Explain the term erythropoiesis.

16.   What is the condition called when the tissues have too little oxygen?

17.   What physiological event is stimulated by hypoxia?

18.   Define the term hematocrit and its relationship to the oxygen-carrying capacity of blood.

19.   What does it mean for an average adult if the Hct is between 0.38 and 0.54?

20.   Correct this statement: The Hct is approximately three times the value of the Hgb.

21.   Explain hemolysis and why it is a serious occurrence.

22.   When hemolysis occurs what problems can a person experience?

6 | White Blood Cells

White blood cells circulate throughout the body and tissues providing protection against foreign organisms and matter. White blood cells are called leukocytes.

leukocytes

To carry out their intended functions, white cells must be highly mobile. They must be able to squeeze through the pores in the capillaries and move into the tissues, a property known as diapedesis. When a foreign organism (referred to as antigen) enters the body, chemical substances are released that stimulate the white cells and cause them to be attracted to the area of invasion. This property is known as chemotaxis.

diapedesis

chemotaxis

Phagocytosis is another property belonging to certain white blood cells, mainly the neutrophils and macrophages. The cell membrane of a phagocyte encloses and internalizes antigen on contact. Once an antigen is internalized, the phagocyte releases powerfully destructive chemicals from its lysosomes (little sacs) that destroy the antigen.

phagocytosis

lysosomes

Figure 6.1 CHEMOTAXIS AND DIAPEDESIS

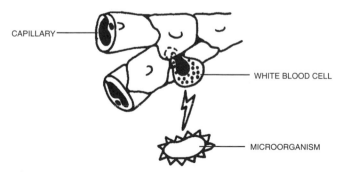

CAPILLARY

WHITE BLOOD CELL

MICROORGANISM

Antigens on the surface of the microorganism release chemicals (chemotaxis) that cause the capillary pores to dilate and allow white blood cells to pass through (diapedesis).

WBCs
1.   2.
Granulocytes   Monocytes
neutrophils   ▼
eosinophils   macrophages
basophils
3.
Lymphocytes
T cells
B cells

White blood cells are divided into three groups: the granulocytes, monocytes, and lymphocytes. Granulocytes are named for the granules present in their cytoplasm, which is the jellylike substance found within the cell. Granulocytes are divided further into neutrophils, eosinophils, and basophils. Monocytes leave the circulatory system and enter the tissues where they become macrophages. The lymphocytes are divided into T cells and B cells. Each white blood cell has a specific response to antigen.

The Number of White Blood Cells

The average adult male has 75 billion circulating white cells. The normal white cell count in a sample of blood from an adult is 4.5-11 x 10^9/L. When an infection occurs in the body the white cell level of the blood increases; for example, to 16 x 10^9/L or higher, depending on the length of time the infection has been present. An increased white cell count is a classic sign of infection somewhere in the body.

Figure 6.2 PHAGOCYTOSIS

WHITE BLOOD CELL

MICRO-   LYSOSOME   WHITE   VACUOLE   LYSOSOME   DIGESTED
ORGANISM   BLOOD   READY   MICRO-
                                CELL   TO RELEASE   ORGANISM
                                ENGULFING   HYDROLYTIC
                                MICRO-   ENZYMES INTO
                                ORGANISM   VACUOLE
                                                                 CONTAINING
                                                                 MICRO-
                                                                 ORGANISM

Granulocytes: Neutrophils, Eosinophils, and Basophils

Neutrophils

NEUTROPHIL

Like other blood cells, neutrophils develop in the hematopoietic marrow. The life cycle of the neutrophil, which takes place in the marrow, blood, and tissues, is short, and in some instances, lasts only a few hours. When neutrophils mature and enter the circulation, 50% of them circulate and 50% adhere to the blood vessel walls. Neutrophils move freely between the blood and tissues of the body where they carry out their primary function of phagocytosis. The surface of neutrophils has receptors for antibody and complement that allow neutrophils to bind to antigens or foreign material coated (opsonized) with antibody or complement.

phagocytosis

In the presence of inflammation or infection, neutrophils, attracted by chemicals, continuously move into the infected area, phagocytize, die, and are themselves phagocytized by macrophages. Neutrophils are generally the first cells to enter an infected area, followed by monocytes.

Eosinophils

EOSINOPHIL

Eosinophils are produced and mature in hematopoietic marrow. They appear at sites where foreign protein and parasites are found and in association with allergic reactions. They make up about 2-5% of the white cells and their numbers increase only slightly in infection, making them difficult to study. Armed with binding sites for IgE and IgG immunoglobulins as well as complement proteins, eosinophils are specifically designed to destroy cells coated with IgG, IgE, and complement. Eosinophils reside in tissues rather than circulate. They live in the skin and the airways (bronchi and bronchioles) of the lungs and release chemicals that damage foreign organisms.

Basophils

BASOPHIL

heparin

histamine

Basophils are produced in the marrow and are the least common of all the granulocytes, making up less than 0.5%. They exhibit chemotaxis and some phagocytic activity. Their main function, it is believed, is to release the anticoagulant heparin in areas of foreign invasion to prevent blood from clotting. If blood clots in the area of invasion, white cells cannot reach the organisms to destroy them and the tissue necroses (dies). Basophils also release histamine, which causes the blood vessels to dilate their pores. Other white blood cells can then leave the circulation more easily and enter the tissues.

Monocytes/Macrophages

MONOCYTE

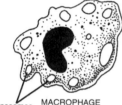

Lysosomes   MACROPHAGE

lysosomes

sinusoids

antigen-presenting cells

Monocytes are produced in the bone marrow and make up about 5% of the circulating white blood cells. They are unlike other blood cells in the circulation because they are immature. When a monocyte leaves the blood it travels to the tissue. Once in the tissue it spends most of its time maturing into a macrophage, while at the same time becoming actively phagocytic. A monocyte has a large horseshoe-shaped nucleus and contains many lysosomes.

As the monocyte develops into a macrophage the number of lysosomes increases. Lysosomes are membrane-bound vacuoles (little sacs found in the cytoplasm of cells) containing enzymes that allow the macrophage to "digest" the foreign matter it engulfs. Macrophages are scattered throughout the body, most commonly lining the sinusoids (spaces) in the liver, spleen, and lungs where they may reside for years available to attack antigen.

Macrophages also circulate throughout the lymphatic system. It is in the lymphatic system that macrophages function as antigen-presenting cells, also called APCs. Antigen-presenting cells are capable of introducing peptide fragments of protein antigens to the T lymphocytes for recognition and destruction. Macrophages play a vital role in the immune response.

Lymphocytes

Lymphocytes are the most complex of the white blood cells and make up about 25% of the circulating white blood cells. Some lymphocytes released from the hematopoietic marrow circulate in the blood while others migrate to the lymph nodes where they wait for antigen. The typical lymphocyte is a small, round cell in which the cytoplasm is almost completely occupied by the nucleus.

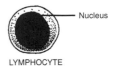

LYMPHOCYTE

The function of the lymphocytes is to generate the immune response when an antigen invades the body. When lymphocytes recognize foreign matter as "not self" they become activated. There are two major types of lymphocytes: the T and B cells. Each type reacts differently to antigen. Within the immune response the T cells release chemicals that activate other white blood cells in responding to antigen. They also release chemicals that lyse antigen. B cells produce antibody.

immune response

T and B cells

antibody

Both T and B lymphocytes retain memory for the offending antigen. Memory lymphocytes can possibly remain in the blood for a lifetime and, therefore, they can respond much faster on subsequent exposure to antigen.

Lymphocytes play a role in the rejection by the body of a transplanted organ. Antigens on the donor organ are recognized by the host lymphocytes as foreign. Host lymphocytes respond and destroy foreign tissue in what is referred to as organ rejection or host-versus-graft disease (HVGD). Conversely, a transplanted organ can be the culprit: its stowaway lymphocytes may recognize the host as foreign and mount an attack against it in a reaction referred to as graft-versus-host disease (GVHD). Graft-versus-host disease can be fatal.

HVGD

GVHD

In both organ rejection and GVHD, similar processes are involved, with the end result being organ failure. Most organ transplant patients must have their immune system suppressed with drugs to prevent organ rejection. An example of an immunosuppressive drug is cyclosporine.

T and B Lymphocytes

receptors

antigen presenting cells

cell-mediated immunity

T cells destroy many types of antigen. After release from hematopoietic marrow, T lymphocytes undergo further maturation in the thymus, a gland that lies on the heart and atrophies with age. The thymus confers on the T cells the ability to recognize antigens as not part of self tissue. The T cell membrane receptors (binding sites for antigen) enable T cells to recognize antigen presented to them by antigen presenting cells. When T cells recognize antigen they initiate the immune response. The role of T cells is to assist other white blood cells (granulocytes, monocytes/macrophages) in reacting to antigen; activate other T cells to become cytotoxic, a property that allows them to lyse antigen; and stimulate B cells to produce antibody specific to a particular antigen. T cell activation by antigen is cell-mediated immunity.

autoimmunity
autoimmune diseases

Usually the T cells in the thymus that recognize and attack self cells are destroyed before they have a chance to harm the body's own tissue. When defective T cells attack self tissue the phenomenon is called autoimmunity. There are many kinds of autoimmune diseases, such as rheumatoid arthritis, diabetes mellitus, and myasthenia gravis.

B cells/plasma cells

humoral immunity

After B cells are released from the hematopoietic marrow most of them reside in the lymph nodes. When B cells recognize antigen or are stimulated by T cells, they differentiate into plasma cells that produce an antibody specific to the offending antigen. Antibody production is enhanced when T cells stimulate B cells. B cells/plasma cells are only involved in antibody production and the only cells in the body capable of producing antibody. Antibody production by B cells/plasma cells is humoral immunity.

Like T cells, B cells can be responsible for autoimmune diseases. Antibodies can attack self tissue, leading to tissue destruction.

Questions

White Blood Cells

1. What is the name of the chemical process that stimulates white cells to the area of foreign invasion? a. diapedesis b. chemotaxis   c. phagocytosis

2. Certain white cells, such as the neutrophils and macrophages, destroy antigen by means of a special property. Name and describe the property.

3. Name the three groups of white blood cells.

4. What does an increased level of white cells indicate?

5. Basophils release two chemicals. Name them.

6. Why is it essential that clotting not take place in an infected area?

7. Explain what happens to monocytes when they leave the blood.

8. What is the role of macrophages in the immune system?

9. Lymphocytes are complex white blood cells. Stimulated by antigens, they produce different types of immune cells. They also initiate immune responses carried out by T and B cells. What role do these cells play in organ transplant rejection?

10. The lymphatic system works in conjunction with the blood-vascular system. How do B cells demonstrate this?

11. How are T cells involved in autoimmune diseases?

7   Plasma

solutes

interstitial fluid

Plasma is the liquid portion of blood in which the formed elements (blood cells) are suspended. It is a straw-colored, viscous solution composed of water and solutes, the latter of which include proteins, lipids, carbohydrates, electrolytes, vitamins, and hormones. The solutes are dissolved in the plasma. They are in continuous communication with the interstitial fluid, which is the fluid that bathes the cells outside the vascular system.

plasma proteins

osmotic/oncotic pressure

Some of plasma's substances, such as proteins, cannot pass easily through the capillary pores due to their large size. The great majority of proteins stay in the vascular space where they exert osmotic pressure, also referred to as oncotic pressure. This pressure maintains fluid (blood volume) in the vascular space because the greater concentration of proteins in capillary blood pulls interstitial fluid from the interstitial space back into the capillary.

buffering

pH of blood

Proteins in plasma perform other functions. They may be used by the tissues when proteins obtained from food do not provide for normal body needs. Along with certain electrolytes, they contribute to the buffering capacity of the blood. Buffering is a term used to describe the body's ability to regulate the pH of blood.

The pH describes the acidity or alkalinity of a solution. If acidic, pH is low, between 1 and 7; if basic, pH is high, between 7 and 14. Numbers 1-7 and 7-14 are logarithmic measurements. The normal range of blood pH is 7.35-7.45, slightly basic.

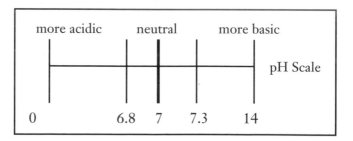

more acidic   neutral   more basic

pH Scale

0   6.8   7   7.3   14

Figure 7.1 FUNCTIONS OF PLASMA

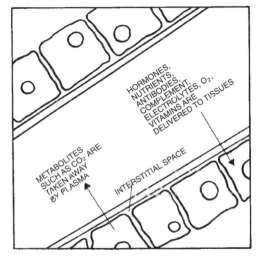

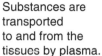

Substances are
transported
to and from the
tissues by plasma.

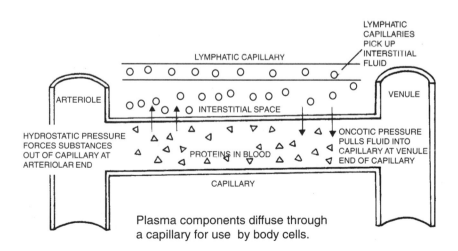

Plasma components diffuse through
a capillary for use by body cells.

acidosis

If the pH of blood changes by becoming either more acidic or basic, there can be serious complications for the patient. For example, in acidosis, carbon dioxide (CO_2) and/or organic acids build up in the blood causing it to become acidic. If acidosis is not corrected, the recovery or health of the patient is compromised because blood and tissue physiology no longer are normal. The lungs and kidneys help control the level of acid.

The Electrolytes and Glucose in Plasma

The electrolytes in plasma have a number of functions. An electrolyte is a chemical molecule that produces ions when placed in a solution such as water or plasma, which is basically water. Normal concentrations of electrolytes are essential for physiologic processes such as nerve conduction, muscle contraction, and blood clotting.

electrolytes

The main electrolytes and their concentrations in plasma are:

Sodium (Na+)   138-148 mM/L*

Potassium (K+)   3.5-5.2 mM/L

Calcium (Ca++)   8.5-10.5 mM/L

Chlorine (Cl-)   98-111 mM/L

The term mMol/L refers to millimoles per liter of solution. The mole is a measure of the molecular weight of a substance.

Calcium, sodium, and potassium are necessary for normal impulse conduction in nerve and muscle fibers. Sodium plays an essential role in maintaining normal fluid balance within the cells of the body. If the sodium concentration is too high or too low, the fluid balance shifts, which means the cells either retain or lose too much fluid.

glucose

Plasma also contains glucose (sugar), an essential source of energy for all tissues of the body. The normal concentration of glucose is 72–137 mg/dL (milligrams per deciliter). Sugar is dissolved in plasma and must get into all cells in order to supply energy. Sugar enters the red blood cell by the simple process of diffusion. Insulin is a hormone produced in the pancreas that allows sugar to penetrate other cells' membranes. Diabetics, people who lack the ability to produce insulin, must take insulin from other sources, such as insulin injection.

diffusion
insulin

The term serum is sometimes used interchangeably with plasma, but the fluids are not the same. When a tube of blood is allowed to stand, the formed elements and coagulation factors form a clot on the bottom of the tube while serum, the straw-colored fluid, rises to the top. Serum is plasma minus the clotting protein fibrinogen. Some blood tests, such as serology tests, routine blood bank tests, and chemistry tests, utilize serum in testing.

serum

fibrinogen

Questions

Plasma

1. What is plasma?

2. Describe two characteristics of plasma.

3. What is the role of solutes in plasma?

4. What is the name of the fluid that bathes cells outside the vascular system? Describe its function.

5. How do plasma proteins maintain fluid in the vascular space?

6. What other functions do plasma proteins provide?

7. The pH of blood is slightly basic. What is the normal range of blood pH?

8. What happens if blood pH becomes either more acidic or more basic?

9. Why are normal concentrations of electrolytes in plasma important in human physiology?

10. What electrolyte in plasma is essential in maintaining normal fluid balance in cells? a. potassium b. calcium c. sodium

11. What is the role of glucose in plasma?

12. Define serum and explain how it is formed from plasma.

8 | Platelets

Platelets, also called thrombocytes, are small, colorless, enucleated bodies. They are produced in the bone marrow by megakaryocytes, which are large cells that produce platelets by fragmenting their cytoplasm. Platelets play a vital role in hemostasis, the prevention of blood loss. When the endothelial lining of a blood vessel is traumatized, platelets are stimulated to go to the site of injury where they form a plug that helps reduce blood loss.

thrombocytes

megakaryocytes

hemostasis

Hemostasis is the process carried out by the body to maintain blood in the vascular system. When blood is lost the body provides platelets and a network of chemicals that prevent additional blood loss by forming a fibrin clot at the site of the damage. Coagulation, also known as blood clotting, is the interaction of platelets with coagulation proteins. The coagulation proteins form fibrin that holds the platelet plug in place.

coagulation

platelet plug

Certain stem cell disorders may cause an increase in platelets, which is a condition called thrombocytosis. Increased bleeding or clotting can occur in thrombocytosis. A decrease in the platelet count is thrombocytopenia. It can be caused by diseases that affect platelet production or by excessive platelet destruction. Thrombocytopenia makes the individual more susceptible to bruising and/or increased bleeding. (See Chapter 12.)

thrombocytosis

thrombocytopenia

Platelets range in size from 2-4 μ, but in certain situations can increase in size. Once platelets are released into the circulatory system they have a life span of 9-12 days. The normal platelet count is 150-450 x 10^9/L for the average adolescent and adult. Young platelets are more effective in achieving and maintaining hemostasis. Old, damaged, and nonfunctional platelets are removed by the spleen.

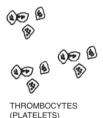

THROMBOCYTES
(PLATELETS)

Questions

Platelets

1. What is another name for platelets?

2. True or false: Platelets are formed elements.

3. Describe the chief function of platelets.

4. What are platelets stimulated to do when the endothelial lining of a blood vessel is damaged?

5. Thrombocytosis is an increase in platelet numbers. What is a decrease called?

6. What conditions can cause an increase or decrease in platelets?

7. What happens to nonfunctional platelets?

8. Define hemostasis and the role of platelets in it.

9 | Hemostasis

The term hemostasis refers to the prevention of blood loss through processes that inhibit blood flow from a ruptured vessel. The hemostatic processes include the following: (1) vascular spasm, (2) platelet function, and (3) blood coagulation (clotting). When a blood vessel is injured or damaged the hemostatic processes repair the break and stop the bleeding.

The first and most immediate hemostatic response to blood vessel injury is vascular spasm, a rapid constriction of small arteries and arterioles. The second response is the formation of a platelet plug. The final response is the initiation of the coagulation cascade, which leads to fibrin production and the formation of a fibrin clot. Together, all the responses help prevent blood loss.

vascular spasm
▼
platelet plug
▼
coagulation cascade
▼
fibrin clot

Once a clot has formed and the vessel has repaired itself, a process known as clot lysis (lysis: to break) must occur so that blood flow through the vessel can resume. Coagulation and clot lysis work in conjunction with each other in achieving hemostasis.

clot lysis

Figure 9.1 MECHANISMS OF COAGULATION

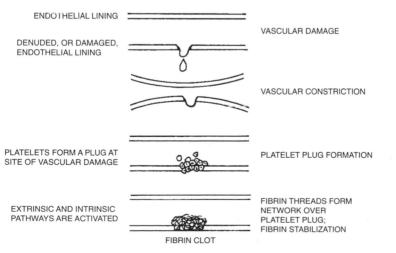

ENDOTHELIAL LINING — VASCULAR DAMAGE

DENUDED, OR DAMAGED, ENDOTHELIAL LINING

VASCULAR CONSTRICTION

PLATELETS FORM A PLUG AT SITE OF VASCULAR DAMAGE — PLATELET PLUG FORMATION

EXTRINSIC AND INTRINSIC PATHWAYS ARE ACTIVATED — FIBRIN THREADS FORM NETWORK OVER PLATELET PLUG; FIBRIN STABILIZATION

FIBRIN CLOT

55

Figure 9.2 MECHANISMS OF PLATELET ACTION

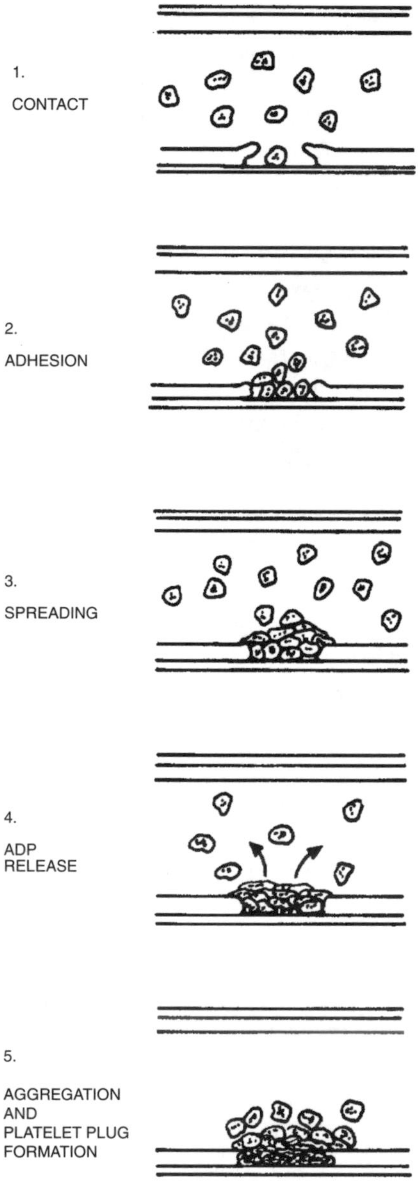

1.

CONTACT

2.

ADHESION

3.

SPREADING

4.

ADP
RELEASE

5.

AGGREGATION
AND
PLATELET PLUG
FORMATION

Vascular Spasm

In vascular spasm the smooth muscle fibers within small arteries and arterioles constrict to reduce the loss of blood. Other events occur in vascular spasm, such as edema (tissue swelling), chemical release, and shunting, which is the redirection of blood flow to nearby vessels.

Arteries and veins have thick walls and cannot control their bleeding by vascular spasm, platelet plug formation, or by coagulation proteins forming a clot. They must be repaired surgically to stop bleeding.

Platelet Function in Coagulation

Platelets perform two functions in coagulation. First, they form a temporary plug that covers the break in the endothelial lining. Second, once the plug is formed, the platelet membrane provides a phospholipid on which the activated coagulation proteins (clotting factors) bind and form a stable fibrin clot. This phospholipid is called platelet factor 3 or PF-3. A phospholipid is a chemically complex fat molecule.

There are five steps involved in platelet plug formation in a damaged vessel. (1) The first step involves contact between the platelets and the damaged endothelial lining of the blood vessel. (2) In the second step, adhesion, the platelets adhere to the damaged surface. (3) Thereafter, the platelets spread out along the damaged surface changing shape (flattening out) as they do. (4) The fourth step is release, in which platelets release a chemical called ADP (adenosine diphosphate). The release of ADP stimulates other platelets to aggregate to the area of damage. (5) The fifth and final step is platelet aggregation.

platelet plug formation
▼
contact
▼
adhesion
▼
spreading
▼
ADP release
▼
aggregation

A platelet plug is formed by the interaction of the above steps, but the plug is only temporary. Coagulation proteins then take up their role to ensure hemostasis by forming a stable fibrin clot.

stable fibrin clot

Prostaglandins that Regulate ADP Release in Platelet Aggregation

thromboxane A₂
prostacyclin

Chemical molecules called prostaglandins regulate ADP by increasing or decreasing the amount of ADP released by platelets. The most important prostaglandins are thromboxane A₂ (TXA_2) and prostacyclin (PGI_2). These molecules work antagonistically in the release of ADP.

ADP

TXA_2 is synthesized in the platelet membrane and increases ADP release thereby ensuring that enough platelets will appear at the site of the injury to form a platelet plug. If not enough platelets go to the site of injury, no plug forms.

PGI_2 is synthesized by the endothelial cells of the vessel wall. This prostaglandin inhibits the platelets from aggregating past the site of damage where they can block blood flow through the vessel. The prostaglandins provide checks and balances in the release of ADP.

Aspirin interferes with normal platelet aggregation. Doctors often prescribe aspirin for patients, as they say, "to help thin the blood." Aspirin does not thin the blood, but it does help reduce the formation of blood clots. Because aspirin blocks the action of TXA_2, it prevents ADP release and therefore platelet aggregation. Neither a platelet plug nor a stable fibrin clot will form. Aspirin therapy aims, for example, at preventing blood clots from forming in the cerebral arteries that can lead to a cerebral vascular accident (CVA, or stroke) and platelets from aggregating in the coronary arteries and causing clot formation (thrombosis). Aspirin is not recommended as a pain reliever following surgery, birth, or anytime the potential for bleeding exists.

Platelet Membrane Phospholipid

phospholipid

Once the platelet plug has formed over the area of injury the coagulation proteins are stimulated to react with a phospholipid released by platelet membranes. Called platelet factor 3 (PF-3), this phospholipid is essential for two reactions in the coagulation cascade.

platelet factor 3

Nature has provided two pathways, the extrinsic and the intrinsic, to prevent bleeding through clot formation. Both fully protect the person from bleeding due either to vessel damage or tissue injury. (See Ch. 10.)

Questions

Hemostasis

1. Explain what vascular spasm, platelet function, and blood coagulation have in common.

2. Which hemostatic process occurs first in hemostasis? Describe what happens.

3. What is the end step in the hemostatic process?

4. For blood flow to resume after a clot has formed, what process must take place?

5. What is the correct version of this statement? Due to their thin walls, arteries and veins can control bleeding by hemostasis and do not need to be repaired surgically.

6. Describe the relationship between platelets and phospholipids.

7. Name the five steps in platelet plug formation.

8. Describe the role of ADP in platelet plug formation.

9. What are the chemicals that regulate ADP release called?

10. Match the correct word – plasma, thromboxane A2, prostacyclin – with the correct statement.

    a. This chemical causes platelets to aggregate to the site of vascular injury.
    b. This chemical inhibits ADP release so platelets do not aggregate past the area of injury.

11. What platelet phospholipid is involved in clotting and when does it become activated?

10 | The Coagulation Cascade

To prevent blood loss a damaged vessel attracts platelets and coagulation factors that form a stable fibrin clot. The coagulation cascade is a complex system of interactions among blood clotting (coagulation) factors that lead to healing of the vessel. The cascade begins when soluble factors are activated to create fibrin, a threadlike protein. Fibrin threads form an insoluble meshwork over the site of the platelet plug and stabilize it. This process is clot formation and the end product of the coagulation cacscade. The prevention of blood loss from a vessel is called hemostasis.

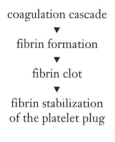

coagulation cascade
▼
fibrin formation
▼
fibrin clot
▼
fibrin stabilization
of the platelet plug

hemostasis

Coagulation factors circulate continuously in the blood and when stimulated by a phospholipid activate one another in the coagulation cascade. The coagulation cascade is initiated by the release of tissue phospholipid (complex fatty acid) from damaged endothelium. Coagulation factors are listed below. The coagulation cascade does not occur in the sequence suggested by the list, however. The factors are referred to by Roman numerals in the order in which they were discovered. Clotting factors are also called clotting proteins or coagulation factors/proteins or serine proteases.

clotting factors are:
coagulation proteins/
coagulation factors
serine proteases

I	Fibrinogen
II	Prothrombin
III	Tissue thromboplastin
IV	Calcium
V	Labile factor (Proaccelerin)
VI	Not assigned
VII	Stable factor (Proconvertin)
VIII	Antihemophilic factor A (AHF)
IX	Christmas factor
X	Stuart-Power factor
XI	Plasma thromboplastin antecedent (PTA)
XII	Hageman factor
XIII	Fibrin stabilizing factor

Factors V, VIII, and XIII are not serine proteases like the other factors. Factors V and VIII are helper factors, or coenzymes. Factors V and VIII are deficient in stored blood. They are preserved, however, in fresh frozen plasma (FFP). Factor XIII is preserved in cryoprecipitate, which is prepared from FFP.

The coagulation cascade involves and is initiated by the activation of the clotting factors. Once a piece of a factor is cleaved (split off), that factor is activated and it then activates the next factor in the cascade. Factors are continually activated until the platelet plug is enmeshed in fibrin.

Clotting factors are produced in the liver and most circulate in the blood in high concentrations in the inactive form. If the proteins were to circulate in the active form, fibrin would form everywhere and the coagulation factors would be very quickly consumed by the body; there would not be enough coagulation factors available for an event requiring coagulation. Because most factors circulate in the inactive form, inappropriate clot formation is minimized.

Blood clots form once the coagulation proteins are activated. Activation depends on the presence of substances not normally present in the blood, such as tissue membrane phospholipid (tissue thromboplastin, or TT), foreign surfaces, and aggregated platelets. In order for coagulation proteins to bind to phospholipids and form a fibrin clot, a normal level of calcium ions (Ca^{++}) must be present in the plasma.

tissue thromboplastin

The release of two phospholipids is required for the formation of a fibrin clot. One is tissue thromboplastin and the other is platelet factor 3 (PF-3). If either phospholipid is unavailable, clot formation will not occur. Tissue thromboplastin is released from damaged cells into the bloodstream and initiates clot formation within the body. PF-3 is found in the platelet membrane and released when platelets aggregate.

platelet factor 3 (PF-3)

Figure 10.1 TRADITIONAL COAGULATION CASCADE

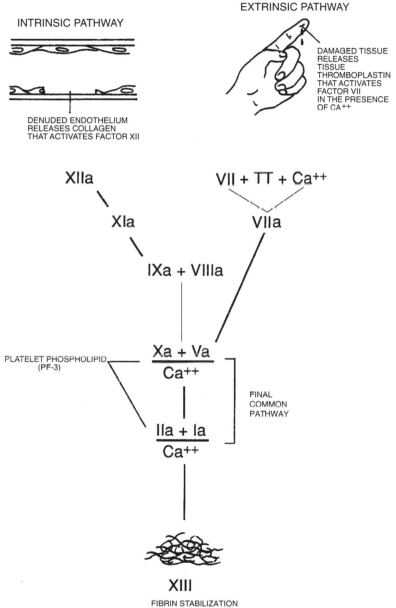

INTRINSIC PATHWAY

EXTRINSIC PATHWAY

DAMAGED TISSUE
RELEASES
TISSUE
THROMBOPLASTIN
THAT ACTIVATES
FACTOR VII
IN THE PRESENCE
OF CA++

DENUDED ENDOTHELIUM
RELEASES COLLAGEN
THAT ACTIVATES FACTOR XII

XIIa

VII + TT + Ca++

XIa

VIIa

IXa + VIIIa

PLATELET PHOSPHOLIPID
(PF-3)

$$\frac{Xa + Va}{Ca^{++}}$$

FINAL
COMMON
PATHWAY

$$\frac{IIa + Ia}{Ca^{++}}$$

XIII

FIBRIN STABILIZATION
OF THE PLATELET PLUG

Ca⁺⁺ bridge

PF-3 is essential for two reactions in the coagulation cascade that take place on the platelet membrane: (1) the activation of factors X and V, and (2) the activation of factors II and I. Phospholipids bind to coagulation factors via a Ca^{++} bridge.

The ability of the body to form clots depends on the availability of clotting factors. If any clotting factor in the cascade is not available, a clot will not form or form too slowly, even if the cascade is initiated. Clotting factor deficiencies occur in diseases in which clotting factors are absent or not replenished, such as hemophilia or liver disease.

The Coagulation Pathways

Theories about blood coagulation are subject to change because new research techniques and more sensitive assays further scientific understanding of this process. In medicine, new findings do not necessarily make traditional theories obsolete; rather, aspects of the traditional may still be considered valid and incorporated into current theory. This holds true for the traditional and current theories of coagulation, both of which are presented in this text.

in vitro
in vivo

Coagulation studies are performed on persons with clotting factor deficiencies and by in vitro (outside the body) experiments. This text focuses on in vivo (within the body) coagulation because different coagulation processes take place in blood that has been removed from the body (in vitro) and in blood within the body.

the intrinsic and extrinsic pathways

In traditional theory the coagulation cascade is described as occurring via two distinct pathways, the intrinsic and extrinsic. The intrinsic pathway is assumed to be the major pathway in the activation of coagulation and the extrinsic a system that functions when the intrinsic fails. By contrast, present theory states that the extrinsic pathway is the major pathway of coagulation whereas the intrinsic pathway plays a minor role and does not initiate coagulation in vivo. In both traditional and current theory, the two pathways are essential for coagulation because individuals with a clotting factor deficiency in either pathway continue to bleed following injury.

The intrinsic pathway is activated by contact with foreign substances; for example, by collagen that is released by damaged blood vessels but not normally present in the blood. Blood exposed to a foreign substance activates factor XII (factor XIIa) and leads to the initiation of the coagulation cascade ("a" means "activated"). Factor XIIa activates factor XI. Factor XIa activates factors IX and VIII. Factors IXa and VIIIa activate factors X and V (start of final common pathway) and is the first set of factors to bind to the platelet phospholipid (PF-3) via Ca^{++}. Factors Xa and Va activate factors II and I, the second reaction involving PF-3 and Ca^{++}. The final common pathway is a point where the enzyme reactions leading to fibrin formation are identical in both pathways.

intrinsic pathway

final common pathway

The extrinsic pathway is activated when damaged tissue releases tissue thromboplastin into the bloodstream; for example, when a vessel is cut. Tissue thromboplastin is a phospholipid extraneous to (not found in) the blood. Factor VII binds to tissue thromboplastin via Ca^{++}, which activates factor VII. Factor VIIa activates factors X and V. Factors Xa and Va activate factors II and I. This point in the pathway is the final common pathway.

extrinsic pathway

Current Theory of In Vivo Coagulation

Current theory regarding coagulation is easier to understand because it removes some of the complexity of the pathways. Although the pathways are still referred to, the focus is on the factors rather than on the interactions of the individual pathways.

The extrinsic pathway initiates in vivo coagulation when tissue thromboplastin (TT) is released into the

Figure 10.2 CURRENT THEORY OF IN VIVO COAGULATION

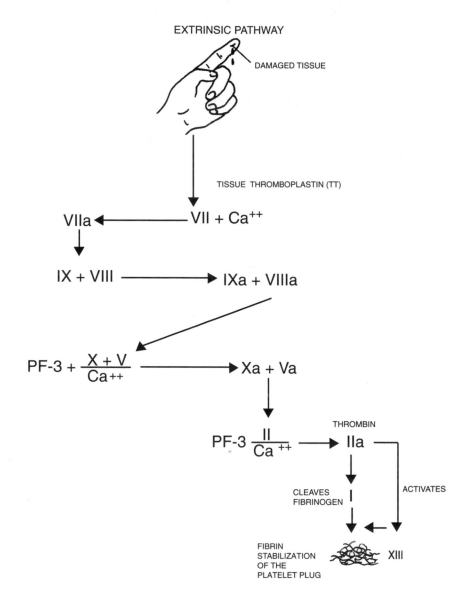

bloodstream from damaged endothelium. It combines with factor VII and Ca^{++} to generate factor VIIa. Factor VIIa activates factors IX and VIII. Factors IXa and VIIIa along with platelet membrane phospholipid (PF-3) and Ca^{++} activate factors X and V. Factors Xa and Va along with Ca^{++} and PF-3 convert prothrombin (factor II) into thrombin (factor IIa).

Thrombin has various functions. For one, it splits fibrinogen (factor I) into small monomers (pieces) of fibrin. The fibrin pieces form a net over the platelet plug. Thrombin also activates factor XIII, which causes the cross-linking of the fibrin threads. Once fibrin threads form a meshwork over the platelet plug, the meshwork stabilizes the clot holding the clot in place (see Fig. 10.2).

thrombin

Present theory regarding coagulation indicates that factors XII and XI have very little, if any, function in coagulation within the body. They are, however, utilized in in vitro coagulation. Factors IX and VIII are activated by factor VIIa rather than by factor XI as in the traditional explanation. Factors IX and VIII are now considered to be the first factors activated in the intrinsic pathway. Factor VIIa does not activate factors X and V as was originally thought but instead activates factors IX and VIII.

Vitamin K and Coumadin™

Vitamin K is a fat-soluble vitamin essential for blood coagulation. Its presence is necessary for liver enzymes to make complete coagulation factors. The coagulation factors that require vitamin K are II, VII, IX, and X.

The drug Coumadin™ (chemical name warfarin) functions as an anticoagulant. It blocks the action of vitamin K-dependent clotting enzymes in the liver. Coumadin™ is not a fast-acting anticoagulant. It must be administered for a few days before the level of the drug is high enough to prevent blood from clotting. Coumadin™ is

anticoagulant

used for the prevention of blood clots, for patients with artificial heart valves, and patients susceptible to strokes.

Clot Lysis

Clot lysis is the dissolution of the blood clot in a healed vessel. It is nature's way of restoring blood flow through a vessel after injury. Clot lysis must occur slowly, for if the clot is dissolved too quickly, before adequate healing takes place, bleeding will resume.

plasminogen

plasmin

TPA

Plasminogen is a naturally occurring enzyme found in the blood. During clot formation, plasminogen is trapped within the clot. After the vessel is healed, plasminogen is cleaved to its active form called plasmin. Plasmin breaks down (lysis) the clot. Plasminogen is activated to plasmin by tissue plasminogen activator (TPA). TPA is a substance produced by tissue cells.

Fibrin Split Products

FSPs

MPS

Kupffer's cells

Small pieces of fibrin are released when a fibrin clot dissolves. They are referred to as fibrin split products (FSPs) or fibrin degradation products (FDPs). Normally FSPs are removed from the circulatory system by a network of cells called the mononuclear phagocytic system (MPS). This network was previously known as the reticuloendothelial system (RES). The cells of the MPS are found throughout the body, but are quite prevalent in the liver where they are referred to as Kupffer's cells.

MPS are phagocytic and remove FSPs from the circulation. If FSPs are not removed from the circulation, they become potent inhibitors of coagulation. They inhibit coagulation by preventing platelets from aggregating and fibrin threads from cross-linking, that is, forming the meshwork of a fibrin clot.

D Dimer assay

The D Dimer assay is used to determine the amount of FSPs in the blood (see Appendix).

Questions

The Coagulation Cascade

1. What is the end product of the coagulation cascade?

2. True or false: The coagulation cascade is like a chain reaction in which coagulation factors are activated to form a fibrin clot.

3. What role do phospholipids have in the coagulation cascade?

4. What are the sources of phospholipids?

5. What would be the consequence if coagulation enzymes circulated in the active form?

6. What are two possible consequences when any one of the clotting factors is not available?

7. Explain the role of calcium in coagulation.

8. Name the two pathways involved in coagulation.

9. True or false: Fibrin production is the result of the activation of both the intrinsic and extrinsic pathways.

10. According to the current theory of coagulation, what is the role of the extrinsic pathway and what is the first factor to be activated?

11. Explain the function of factor XII in in vivo coagulation.

12. Explain the role of vitamin K in blood coagulation.

13. Define clot lysis and explain its importance to the resumption of blood flow.

14. What is the role of TPA in clot dissolution?

15.   Name the assay that evaluates the presence of FSPs in the blood.

16.   How are fibin split products (FSPs) removed from the body?

17.   If FSPs were to remain in circulation, what would happen with respect to coagulation?

18.   What organ synthesizes most of the clotting factors?

19.   Why is coagulation essential to hemostasis?

11 | Coagulation System Disorders

Coagulation system disorders may cause increased bleeding or increased clotting, depending on the disorder. For example, in a thrombotic disorder there is an increase in blood clot formation within the body. Most coagulation factor disorders cause increased bleeding and are referred to as hemorrhagic.

thrombotic

hemorrhagic

Loss of Vascular Integrity

Vascular integrity refers to the natural state of vessels that allows blood to flow through in an uninterrupted fashion. Any time a blood vessel is injured, whether as a result of surgery or other cause, blood flow is interrupted and vascular integrity is lost.

Blood vessel abnormalities can lead to loss of vascular integrity. The abnormalities may be due to either congenital or acquired defects. An example of a congenital defect is Marfan's syndrome, which causes arterial walls to weaken, making them susceptible to rupture. Death may result. An example of an acquired defect is atherosclerosis (plaque buildup in arteries). Both congenital and acquired defects may require surgery to control bleeding.

Coagulation Factor Disorders

When a coagulation factor is deficient, bleeding occurs because fibrin stabilization of the platelet plug cannot take place. Coagulation pathways are assessed by testing a sample of the patient's blood. (See Appendix.)

There are many types of coagulation protein deficiencies. They may be congenital or acquired. A congenital factor deficiency, such as hemophilia, involves a single protein abnormality, lasts for a person's lifetime, and is rare. Acquired factor deficiencies are different from hereditary disorders in that they involve multiple factors and are common. Examples are liver disease and vitamin K defi-

congenital factor deficiency

acquired factor deficiency

71

ciency. Usually, with an acquired factor deficiency a sudden onset of bleeding occurs.

Disseminated Intravascular Coagulation

Disseminated intravascular coagulation (DIC) is a pathologic disorder that activates the hemostatic system and is characterized by bleeding. Many medical conditions, diseases, and disorders referred to as "triggering events" can lead to DIC. Triggering events initiate widespread fibrin (clot) formation and clot lysis in a diffuse, uncontrolled manner throughout the body's vasculature. Triggering events inititate DIC by releasing tissue thromboplastin or similar substances into the bloodstream. DIC can follow widespread endothelial damage or platelet aggregation.

Clotting consumes large amounts of platelets and coagulation factors, the depletion of which causes the bleeding associated with DIC. Clot lysis (breakdown) produces fragments called fibrin split products (FSPs) that further interfere with coagulation because they inhibit platelet aggregation and the cross-linking of fibrin threads. Blood clot formation within the microvasculature causes blockage (thrombosis) of the capillaries leading to tissue necrosis and/or organ dysfunction.

Causes

The following conditions, disorders, and diseases can act as triggering events for DIC: (1) obstetrical complications, such as amniotic fluid embolus and retained placenta; (2) malignancies, such as some leukemias and solid organ malignancies; (3) infectious organisms, such as gram-negative bacteria and viruses; (4) widespread tissue damage, such as burns and crush injuries; (5) vascular malformations, such as vascular tumors and aortic aneurysm; (6) immunologic disorders, such as anaphylactic and allergic reactions, as well as immune complexes; (7) the release of toxins by certain bacteria or the release of cytokines in response to infection; (8)

triggering events

tissue necrosis
organ dysfunction

pieces of particulate matter, such as red cell stroma from hemolyzed red blood cells; and (9) some snake and spider venoms. There are other triggering events as well.

Complications associated with DIC include tissue necrosis and organ dysfunction due to thrombosis in the microvasculature in the kidneys, brain, and lungs. Hemorrhage is also a complication. It is caused by decreased levels of platelets, coagulation factors, and increased amounts of FSPs in the blood. Red blood cell hemolysis occurring in the microvasculature is common in DIC. Hemolysis further increases clotting by releasing tissue thromboplastin into the bloodstream.

hemorrhage

Signs and Symptoms

The signs and symptoms of the triggering event, such as retained placenta, are usually obvious. Occasionally the signs and symptoms are not obvious, such as those associated with certain rare malignancies. All severely ill patients should be evaluated for DIC. Usually the sicker the patient the more severe the DIC is. Ill newborns have increased chances of developing DIC because their body systems are immature and incapable of responding to the complications of DIC. Pregnant women at full term (9 months) are susceptible to DIC because they have increased levels of circulating coagulation proteins, that is, they are hypercoaguable.

In children, DIC is most often caused by burns, infections, and trauma. Adults usually develop DIC in association with malignancies and infections.

The most common sign of DIC is bleeding usually manifested as skin discoloration due to hemorrhage (bleeding) into the tissues. Continued bleeding from either traumatic or surgical wounds is another sign of DIC. Bleeding occurs as a result of decreased levels of platelets and coagulation factors, especially factor V, prothrombin (factor II), and fibrinogen (factor I). Bleeding also can be due to the increased amounts of FSPs within the circulation.

factor V

prothrombin (factor II)

fibrinogen (factor I)

Diagnosis

The lab tests used in diagnosing DIC are the prothrombin time (PT), thrombin time (TT), activated partial thromboplastin time (aPTT), platelet count (PC), fibrinogen level, and the D Dimer assay that measures the level of fibrin split products (FSPs).

Lab results can vary depending on the triggering event. For example, lab test results from hypoxic individuals can show a normal platelet count and fibrinogen level, a slightly prolonged PT, and increased levels of FSPs. Bacterial and viral infections can present quite different results, such as a low platelet count, increased levels of FSPs, decreased fibrinogen, slightly increased PT, and a normal aPTT.

Management

The management of DIC is problematic because physicians have different theories about how it should be treated. However, there is agreement that treating and resolving the triggering event is the first essential step. The blood components selected are determined by the results of the lab tests.

To restore hemostasis in individuals with DIC, cryoprecipitate, platelets, and fresh frozen plasma are administered to replenish depleted clotting factors and platelets. If shock and low blood volume are evident, fresh frozen plasma is administered to replenish volume, clotting factors, and the oncotic effect of plasma proteins. Pharmacologic therapies for treating DIC include (1) heparin, which is used occasionally but is controversial because it potentiates bleeding; (2) specific factor replacements, such as protein C and antithrombin III; and (3) antifibrinolytics, the use of which is also controversial.

Questions

Coagulation System Disorders

1. True or false: All coagulation disorders cause bleeding to occur.

2. What is meant by vascular integrity and when is it lost?

3. Describe two causes of the loss of vascular integrity.

4. Why does bleeding occur when there are defective coagulation factors?

5. What is the difference between a congenital and an acquired coagulation deficiency?

6. Name the two chief events in DIC.

7. What are two causes of DIC?

8. What physiological event occurs when surfaces are denuded of endothelium?

9. What blood components are consumed during DIC?

10. Until the cause of DIC is discovered, what must be done for the patient?

11. When FSPs are released in the circulation, clot formation is inhibited. If the FSP concentration is high enough, what happens to platelets?

12 | Platelet Disorders

Platelet disorders can involve either the quality or quantity of platelets. Quality refers to the ability of platelets to form a platelet plug and quantity to the number of platelets in the circulation.

Two tests are used to determine the cause of a bleeding disorder. The bleeding time tests platelet quality and the platelet count the quantity. (See Appendix.)

Platelet Quality

When platelet quality is poor, platelets may not be able to adhere to or aggregate at the site of endothelial damage. Platelet quality can be affected by various drugs, such as aspirin, protamine, heparin, and dextran. Also affecting platelet quality are conditions such as liver disease, von Willebrand's disease, defects due to storage, and high concentrations of fibrin split products. Patients with poor platelet quality are treated with transfusions of platelets.

Platelet Quantity

thrombocytopenia

A low platelet count is referred to as thrombocytopenia. An individual is considered to have thrombocytopenia when the platelet count is less than 150 x 10 ^{9}/L, a number that applies to all age groups. Someone with a low platelet count experiences an increase in bleeding because not enough platelets are available to form a platelet plug. There are many causes of thrombocytopenia. A transfusion of platelets is the usual means of treating patients with a low platelet count.

Conditions causing a low platelet count include massive blood loss, bone marrow tumors, radiation or chemotherapy, and the formation of antibodies to platelets (the immune response). A significant cause of a low platelet count can be the massive consumption of platelets in the formation of clots. DIC is an example. The bone marrow reserve of platelets is limited and can be quickly depleted following blood loss or platelet destruction.

A platelet count greater than 450 x 10⁹/L is referred to as thrombocytosis. This condition may cause increased bleeding or increased clot formation. Thrombocytosis is usually due to a disease of the bone marrow. Treatment is aimed at reducing the number of platelets, usually by means of chemotherapeutic agents.

thrombocytosis

Questions

Platelet Disorders

1. Platelet disorders can involve the quality or quantity of platelets. What is meant by the quality of platelets?

2. What test is used to determine whether a bleeding disorder is due to the quantity of platelets? The quality?

3. Match the terms with the correct phrases: a. thrombocytopenia b. thrombocytosis

   A platelet count less than 150 x 10^9/L

   A platelet count more than 450 x 10^9/L

4. Describe a manifestation of poor platelet quality.

5. Cite two causes of a low platelet count.

6. Cite two causes of poor platelet quality.

7. What happens to platelets in DIC?

8. What is the main cause of thrombocytosis?

13 | Blood Transfusion

Blood transfusion is the infusion of blood or blood components into patients for treating a variety of surgical and medical conditions. Also called transfusion therapy, it involves one of the following: allogeneic (someone else's) blood, autologous (one's own) blood, or any blood component or its substitutes. Blood is a living tissue, therefore, a transfusion of whole blood or any of its components from one individual to another can be considered a transplant, just like a kidney, heart, or liver transplant. A blood transfusion is given to replace blood lost during trauma or surgery, to treat anemia, hemophilia, and internal bleeding, and to replace a specific blood component destroyed by chemotherapy.

transfusion therapy
allogeneic blood
autologous blood
blood component

Before the discovery of blood groups in the early part of this century, blood transfusion was hazardous; it was successful only by chance. Over time the risks of disease transmission and transfusion reaction have been greatly reduced.

Before blood components can be transfused, certain steps must be followed. Whole blood is collected from a donor or patient in a blood bag containing an anticoagulant/preservative. It is usually processed into components, such as packed red cells, platelets, and plasma. All blood is grouped and cross matched for compatibility to prevent transfusion reactions. Blood and blood components are tested for diseases and stored according to blood group and other criteria. They are then available for transfusion. During a transfusion the patient must be monitored for a possible transfusion reaction.

Blood Donation

Blood donation is the collection of blood or blood components from individuals for use in transfusions. Blood from a donor is called allogeneic, and from one's self autologous. Any adult free of a serious disease or medical condition may donate blood. Certain conditions and diseases prevent a person from donating, however. These include pregnancy; anemia, which is a low red blood cell count; a history of malaria, which is a blood disease transmitted by the mosquito; a history of hepatitis, which is a disease affecting the liver; heart disease; and infection with the immunodeficiency virus (HIV). Eligible adults may donate blood once every 8 weeks.

A candidate for blood donation is given extensive medical questioning and a basic physical screening that includes temperature, pulse, blood pressure, Hct (0.38) and Hgb (12.5 g/dL). As long as the results of the medical screening are acceptable, donation can begin.

Figure 13.1 BLOOD DONATION SET

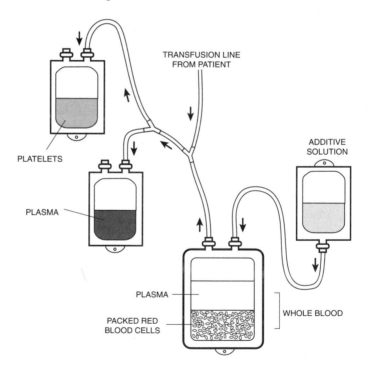

Blood is usually withdrawn through veins in the crux of the elbow. A tourniquet is tightened around the upper arm to cause the veins to bulge to make the insertion of a large-bore needle easier. The needle is connected to a blood bag containing an anticoagulant/preservative, which can be CPD, CP2D, or CPDA-1. These solutions are added to maintain red cell viability,help maintain blood pH, and to prevent clotting. As the blood enters the bag, it mixes with the anticoagulant/preservative.

Approximately 1 pint of whole blood, 450 mL, is collected in a typical donation. A pint represents about 1/10 of the donor's total blood volume. Whole blood contains all the components of blood.

whole blood

After whole blood is collected, it is usually processed into its various components for storage and later use. The blood is tested for various antigenic markers for hepatitis B and C, HTLV-I/II (human T cell lymphotropic virus), and HIV. Blood is also tested for the bacterium that causes syphilis. If the tests are negative, the blood components can be used for transfusions.

The Citrate Anticoagulants/Preservatives: CPD, CP2D, and CPDA-1

CPD, CP2D, and CPDA-1 are known collectively as the citrate anticoagulants/preservatives. They are commercially prepared solutions used only in the collection and storage of blood and blood components for transfusion. The solutions are placed in blood bags by the manufacturer and have two functions: (1) to prevent collected blood from clotting and (2) to provide nutrients for preserving and maintaining the viability of the red blood cells. Blood would clot within minutes if CPD, CP2D, or CPDA-1 were not used in collection. Anticoagulants/preservatives are used in the collection of whole blood, after which packed red cells, platelets, and plasma are then prepared.

red blood cell viability

The solutions CPD, CP2D and CPDA-1 contain the chemicals citrate, phosphate, and dextrose. CPDA-1 contains adenine. CP2D contains twice the amount of dextrose as the other solutions. The "C" in CPD, CP2D, and CPDA-1 stands for citrate. Citrate is the anticoagulant; the other chemicals are the preservatives.

citrate

phosphate

ATP

dextrose

adenine

The chemicals in anticoagulants/preservatives have special functions. Citrate prevents clotting by binding the calcium (Ca^{++}) dissolved in the blood plasma and normally used in coagulation. Phosphate helps prevent pH changes and maintain normal levels of adenosine triphosphate (ATP) in the blood. ATP is a high-energy compound produced in a cellular organelle called the mitochondria and is an energy source for most cellular reactions. The chemical reaction between glucose and oxygen in the cell produces ATP. High levels of ATP in red cells permit better oxygen delivery to the tissues. Dextrose, also known as glucose, is a simple sugar that helps to maintain red blood cell viability. The chemical adenine in CPDA-1 aids the red blood cell in maintaining high levels of ATP. Except for citrate, all the chemicals in the solutions aid in maintaining and extending the storage life of the red blood cell.

Whole blood collected in CPD and CP2D can be refrigerated for 21 days and 35 days when collected in CPDA-1. Whole blood and packed red cells are stored at 1-6C. Other components require different storage temperatures.

Additive Systems

After blood has been collected and the blood bag is full, most of the plasma is removed from the unit, either by centrifugation (spinning down) or by the effect of gravity.

packed red cells

Once the plasma has been removed, packed red cells remain, along with minimal amounts of platelets, plasma, and white blood cells. A clear liquid referred to as an additive system is usually added to packed red cells to increase their storage shelf life.

An additive system of 100 mL may be added to a unit of packed red cells. It must be added within 72 hours of collection. Additive systems increase storage shelf life from the time of collection to 42 days. They help the red blood cells carry on their normal metabolic processes. When additive systems are to be used, CPD is usually the anticoagulant in which whole blood is collected.

Additive systems is the generic name for commercially prepared chemical solutions that contain adenine, dextrose, saline, and mannitol. These chemicals aid only in the preservation of red blood cells; they have no anticoagulative properties. There are three commercially prepared solutions recommended by the FDA. They are added only to packed red blood cells.

Blood Banking

Blood banks are operated by hospitals, the Red Cross, and private facilities. Blood and blood components are banked (stored) according to standards established by the American Association of Blood Banks (AABB). Each component is stored according to the time and temperature required for maintaining its viability. Blood and blood components are available from blood banks for patients as needs arise. For example, platelets are ready for patients actively bleeding due to thrombocytopenia or abnormal platelets and plasma components are ready for patients with bleeding disorders such as liver disease

AABB

Whole blood, packed red cells, and platelets are organized in blood banks by the ABO/Rh systems. All units of blood are labeled by blood group – A+, B-, AB+, and so on – to ensure that right blood and component can be selected.

ABO/Rh

Defects in Banked Blood

The longer blood is stored the less viable its components become, a condition called storage lesion. Whole blood more than 24 hours old has few viable platelets and white blood cells. A decrease in the levels of clotting factors V and VIII also occurs. Due to their short shelf life, these factors are called the labile factors. Other clotting factors maintain their levels of activity during storage and are called the stable factors.

storage lesion

labile factors

stable factors

Over time, all stored units of blood suffer damage, which is a natural occurrence. Blood is a living tissue and must have a favorable environment to carry out cellular metabolism and maintain its viability.

Blood Grouping and Cross Matching

blood grouping

cross matching

All blood belongs to one of four groups (A, B, AB, O) in the ABO system. Identification of the donor and recipient's ABO and Rh blood groups is called blood grouping. Determining that there is compatibility between a specific donor and recipient is known as cross matching. Blood grouping and cross matching tests must be performed before transfusions can be administered.

forward typing

reverse typing

reagent

Donor and recepient blood groups are identified by forward (cell) and reverse (serum) typing tests. Forward typing determines the presence or absence of A and B antigens on the red cell membrane. The testing laboratory uses reagent anti-A and anti-B antibodies to determine the antigens. Reverse typing determines the antibodies present in the serum. Reagent red blood cells known to have group A or B antigens are mixed with either donor or recipient serum. A reagent is a strong concentration of antibodies or red cells prepared by manufacturers.

agglutination
hemolysis

If an agglutination reaction and/or hemolysis occurs in either the forward or reverse typing test, the laboratory

Figure 13.2 CROSS MATCHING

I = Incompatible
C= Compatible

To determine blood compatibility for transfusion purposes, recipient serum (plasma minus fibrinogen) is mixed with the red cells of various donors. If the cells do not clump, a donor's blood can be mixed with the recipient's blood in a transfusion.

RECIPIENT BLOOD GROUP

DONOR BLOOD GROUP (PACKED RED CELLS ONLY)	O	A	B	AB
O	C	C	C	C
A	I	C	I	C
B	I	I	C	C
AB	I	I	I	C

can then determine the blood group. For example, if agglutination of red blood cells occurs when serum is mixed with reagent cells carrying the A antigen, the serum contains anti-A antibody. This tells medical personnel that the serum is from a group B or O individual. The Rh antigen on the red cell is determined in the same way and at the same time.

In cross matching, donor red cells and recipient serum are mixed. This test looks for antibodies in the recipient's serum that agglutinate or hemolyze donor red cells. If the red cells agglutinate or hemolyze on the microscope slide, the donor and recipient have incompatible blood. The absence of agglutination or hemolysis indicates compatible blood.

Filtering of Blood

All blood products, except commercially prepared ones, should be transfused through a blood filter before infusion into the patient. Blood filters filter out particulate matter such as hemolyzed red cells, cell fragments, plastic debris, and blood clots that may have formed during collection or storage. Some filters remove formed elements, specifically the white blood cells.

Blood filters are available in many sizes. Standard blood filters have pore sizes of 170-260 μ. Microaggregate filters have smaller pore sizes (20-40 μ) and trap microaggregate (tiny) particles such as pieces of fibrin, fragments of platelets, and white cells. Filters are placed in the intravenous (I.V.) line between the bag and the patient.

microaggregate filters

Filters that remove white blood cells from blood and blood components are called leukocyte-adsorption filters or leukocyte-depletion filters. Units of packed red cells and platelets contain small amounts of white cells. These cellular components must be removed before transfusion to certain patients, who, as a result of multiple transfusions, react to the major histocompatibility/human leukocyte antigen on the membrane of the white cells (MHC/HLA). The MHC/HLA antigen cannot be removed from the membrane: the white cells must be filtered out.

leukocyte-adsorption
leukocyte-depletion
filters

A unit of blood may be filtered either before storage or at the bedside. It is preferable to remove white cells before storage, when they are intact. During storage many of them become fragmented, making removal more difficult.

Blood Administration

Before a transfusion can begin, medical personnel must confirm that the identification numbers on the blood bag match those on the patient's chart. The correct blood group must be given to the patient. Medication is never added to a blood bag and all blood and blood components should be filtered before transfusion. During transfusion the patient's vital signs (pulse, blood pressure, temperature) are taken regularly for any possible sign of a transfusion reaction.

tubing set

In preparation for a transfusion a needle is inserted into the vein. The blood administration set, also called a tubing set, is attached to the needle. The tubing set has either a single

Figure 13.3 BLOOD ADMINISTRATION SET

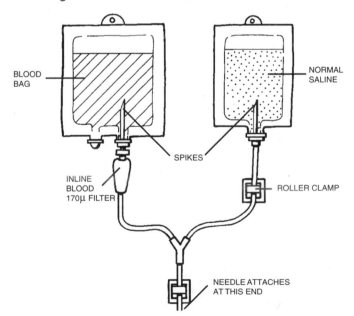

BLOOD BAG

NORMAL SALINE

SPIKES

INLINE BLOOD 170μ FILTER

ROLLER CLAMP

NEEDLE ATTACHES AT THIS END

or double spike. Each tubing set comes with a 170 μ filter in place. The double-spike set allows units of blood and saline or albumin to be infused at the same time. All air in the tubing line must be expressed before the needle is inserted into the vein to begin the transfusion. Air is expressed from the intravenous (I.V.) line by opening the roller clamp and running the blood or blood product plus saline (if necessary) into the I.V. line until the blood exits from the needle. The I.V. line runs from the blood bag to the needle into the vein.

Normal saline is a salty solution that helps reduce the viscosity of blood or blood product so that it flows more freely. A unit of normal saline is attached to the I.V. line and infused along with the blood. Normal saline is always the solution of choice when transfusing blood or blood components. It does not damage the cells as do other I.V. solutions. For example, dextrose causes hemolysis and lactated Ringer's increases Ca^{++}, which may cause the blood to clot.

normal saline

Questions

Blood Transfusion

1. Define blood transfusion and two situations in which it may be required.

2. What is the difference between autologous and allogeneic blood?

3. List the steps involved in preparing whole blood for transfusion purposes.

4. Identify three persons who may not donate blood.

5. What steps are taken to determine the eligibility of an adult to donate blood?

6. The hemoglobin concentration of a blood donor must be at a certain level. What is the level?

7. How much donor blood is collected in a typical donation?

8. Why are CPD, CP2D, and CPDA-1 placed in blood bags? What is the term that refers to these solutions?

9. What is citrate and explain its function in CPD, CP2D, and CPDA-1?

10. CPDA-1 contains adenine. What role does this chemical have in maintaining the viability of red blood cells?

11. What is the storage life of whole blood and packed red cells collected in CPD and CP2D? In CPDA-1?

12. Explain when and why and approximately how much additive system is added to packed red cells. Include a definition of additive system in the answer.

13. Why do blood banks store whole blood, packed cells, and platelets according to the ABO/Rh systems?

14. Describe what happens to blood the longer it is stored.

15. Why must blood grouping and cross matching be done before a transfusion can be administered?

16. How are reagents used to determine blood groups?

17. What does forward typing determine? Reverse typing?

18. a. What blood group is indicated if agglutination occurs when reagent B cells are mixed with serum?

    b. What blood group is indicated if no agglutination occurs when red blood cells are added to serum containing anti-A and anti-B antibodies?

19. In cross matching, which is determined, (a) blood group or (b) compatibility between blood groups?

20. All noncommercial blood products should be filtered before a transfusion. Cite three examples of particulate matter that filters trap.

21. What is the name of the filter that traps white cells, and why must this filter be used?

22. True or false: Medication is never added to a blood bag.

23. Give two reasons why normal saline is administered along with blood in a transfusion.

Transfusion Reactions

There are many different kinds of transfusion reactions, including hemolytic, febrile (nonhemolytic), and allergic. They vary in severity and number of symptoms. A reaction can occur as the result of an incompatible ABO/Rh transfusion or patient sensitization to transfused white cells, platelets, or plasma proteins. (See Chart 4, p. 94.)

hemolytic transfusion
A, B, Rh antigens

A hemolytic transfusion reaction occurs when donor and recipient blood groups are incompatible. A, B, or Rh antigens on the red blood cell membrane of the donor react to, or are incompatible with, the antibodies in the recipient's plasma. Anti-A, anti-B, or Rh antibodies in the recipient's plasma cause the donor red cells to hemolyze (burst). Hemolysis of the red blood cell membrane releases hemoglobin (Hgb) into the plasma. Plasma-free hemoglobin is hemoglobin that has left the red cell and entered the plasma. Group O blood has no antigens, therefore, there is usually no transfusion reaction.

hemolysis

plasma-free hemoglobin

Figure 14.1 RED CELL LYSIS DUE TO A TRANSFUSION REACTION

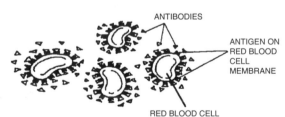

ANTIBODIES

ANTIGEN ON
RED BLOOD
CELL
MEMBRANE

RED BLOOD CELL

In an incompatible transfusion reaction, antibodies in the recipient's plasma attach to the antigens on the red blood cell membrane.

When the antibodies attach to the antigen a transfusion reaction occurs. Rupturing of the red blood cell membrane releases hemoglobin (Hgb) into the plasma, which becomes plasma-free Hgb.

HGB RELEASED FROM
RUPTURED RED BLOOD CELL

An immediate life-threatening situation can develop in an incompatible ABO blood transfusion.

A hemolytic transfusion reaction can include some or all of the following symptoms: reddening of the face (flushing), an increased rate of breathing (hyperventilation), an increased heart rate (tachycardia), a sense of fright, patchy blotches of skin (urticaria), shortness of breath (dyspnea), chest pressure, and back pain. A feeling of nausea may occur and, in some instances, progress to vomiting. Cyanosis (bluish color to skin) and fever in the range of 102-105F may be evident. Severe back pain in a transfusion reaction is caused by hemolyzed red cell membranes that activate the clotting mechanism. Clots block the microvasculature (capillaries) of the kidneys. Blockage of the microvasculature can cause renal failure.

The most feared incompatible blood transfusion reaction is renal failure, the delayed complication caused by hemolysis. This event can be triggered even when only a small amount of incompatible ABO blood is administered. When renal shutdown does occur the patient is slowly poisoned because the kidneys cannot remove impurities from the blood. Dialysis usually is required to cleanse the blood. The dialysis procedure is performed 2 or 3 times a week or until kidney function returns to normal.

renal failure

There is almost always some renal tubular necrosis (damage to the tubules in the kidney) when large amounts of ABO-incompatible blood are infused. In certain patients, the condition is irreversible and damage to the kidney is permanent – another essential reason to type and cross match donor red cells and recipient serum.

renal tubular necrosis

Chart 1: Common Signs and Symptoms of a Transfusion Reaction

Signs and symptoms:

- Fever and chills
- Chest and back pain
- Sore aching muscles
- Headache
- Numbness and tingling
- Pain at infusion site
  (needle puncture site)
- Wheezing and coughing
- Dyspnea (shortness of breath)
- Tachypnea (increased rate of breathing)
- Stomach cramps and diarrhea
- Nausea and vomiting
- Increase or decrease of blood pressure
- Irregular heartbeat
- Flushing of the skin (reddening)
- Cyanosis (blue coloring)
- Edema (swelling)
- Changes in amount of urine;
  either increase or decrease
- Dark color to urine
- Renal failure
- Bleeding
- Urticaria (rash and hives)
- Sweating

**Chart 2: Steps to Follow When the Signs and Symptoms
of a Transfusion Reaction Occur**

- Stop the transfusion immediately
- Maintain an I.V. of 0.9% normal saline to maintain venous access for drug administration
- Report the incident to physician and blood bank
- Check the blood bag identification numbers with those in the patient chart
- Treat symptoms appropriately
- Send the unused portion of blood in the blood bag and the administration set to the blood bank
- Collect and send blood and urine samples to the laboratory
- Document the transfusion reaction and treatment thoroughly

**Chart 3: Transfusion Reaction in the Unconscious or
Anesthetized Patient**

Signs and symptoms:

- Weak or absent pulse
- Decrease in blood pressure
- Small amount of urine, possibly none, produced
- Fever
- Increase or decrease in the heart rate
- Increase in the amount of bleeding during surgery
- Visible signs of Hgb in the urine (hemoglobinuria)

Actions:

Stop the transfusion immediately and monitor the patient closely
Initiate treatment

Chart 4: Transfusion Reactions

Acute Hemolytic
Description: A serious life-threatening reaction
Causes: A transfusion of ABO incompatible blood, packed cells, or components. Antibodies in recipient plasma attach to the transfused red blood cells, leading to lysis of the transfused red blood cells.
Signs and Symptoms: See Chart 1. Patients can experience many of the serious complications such as renal failure, shock, pulmonary edema, DIC, and hemolysis.
Actions: Stop the transfusion immediately. Monitor the patient closely.

Anaphylactic Shock
Description: One of the most severe transfusion reactions. It occurs in individuals who have developed antibodies to certain antigens.
Causes: Transfusion of blood components, plasma, and certain drugs such as penicillin
Signs and Symptoms: Coughing, bronchospasm, laryngeal, edema, shock
Actions: Attend to immediately. This is a full-blown medical emergency.

Circulatory Overload
Description: Similar to congestive heart failure or pulmonary edema
Causes: A transfusion of fluid into a patient faster than his or her circulatory system can accommodate
Signs and Symptoms: Pulmonary edema, shortness of breath
Actions: Eliminate excess fluid from the body by means of diuretics

continued

Chart 4 *continued*

Mild allergic
Description: Usually a relatively mild reaction
Causes: Sensitization to foreign plasma proteins of the donor
Signs and Symptoms: See Chart 2. Patients can experience some of the milder transfusion reactions, e.g., uticaria, headache, dizziness. This reaction rarely progresses to more serious complications.
Actions: Watch the patient for other more serious complications.

Sepsis
Description: Usually not a problem, depending on the bacterial contaminant
Causes: Transfusion of contaminated blood or blood components
Signs and Symptoms: See Chart 1. Patients can experience high fever, chills, diarrhea, vomiting, hypotension, and shock.
Actions: Take blood cultures from the recipient and administer appropriate antibiotics. Monitor the patient closely.

Febrile, nonhemolytic
Description: The most common reaction following a blood transfusion
Causes: Sensitization to antigens on the white blood cells, platelets, or plasma proteins of the donor
Signs and Symptoms. See Chart 1. Patients can experience nonlife-threatening signs and symptoms such as fever, headache, and chills. This reaction rarely progresses to more serious complications.
Actions: Treat symptoms as necessary

Questions

Transfusion Reactions

1. What is a transfusion reaction?

2. True or false: Group AB blood has both A and B antigens on the red cell membrane and can cause a transfusion reaction if given to a person with group B.

3. What happens to hemoglobin when a red blood cell is hemolyzed?

4. True or false: An ABO incompatible transfusion reaction can be fatal.

5. Describe five signs and symptoms of a hemolytic transfusion reaction.

6. Renal failure is a complication of a severe transfusion reaction and can lead to the death of a patient. Explain why.

7. What is the first step that must be taken by a health care worker during a transfusion reaction?

8. Name three types of acute transfusion reactions. Refer to Chart 4, p. 94.

15 | Transfusion and Disease Transmission

During the 1980s the fear of contracting AIDS forced the public and medical community to question the safety of allogeneic blood and blood products. Several developments have greatly reduced the incidence of all disease transmission by transfusion: newly developed blood tests, which are approximately 99% accurate; more stringent standards applied to donors; and permission extended to donors to self-exclude anonymously. Nevertheless, diseases transmitted by transfusion remain a threat to recipients. Hepatitis, which is potentially fatal, and AIDS, which is usually fatal, are two viral diseases of major concern to patients and health care professionals.

The testing of blood and blood components is required by the American Association of Blood Banks (AABB) and the Food and Drug Administration (FDA). These organizations set the standards for all blood banking and transfusion policies in the United States. All blood donations are screened for certain transmissible bacterial and viral diseases. The tests detect either antigen or antibodies against microorganisms. Blood that contains either antigen or antibodies to microorganisms is seropositive. Seronegative blood shows no evidence of disease.

AABB
FDA

seropositive
seronegative

All blood must be tested for hepatitis B and C, which are viruses affecting the liver; elevated levels of alanine aminotransferase (ALT), which may indicate hepatitis (this test was discontinued); human immunodeficiency viruses 1 and 2 (HIV 1/2); human T cell lymphotropic virus (HTLV-1/II), a viral precursor to leukemia, lymphoma, and a paralytic disease that affects the nervous system; and syphilis, which is caused by a bacterium.

hepatitis B and C

HIV 1/2
HTLV-1/II
syphilis

If a donor's blood tests positive for any of the above diseases, the blood is discarded and the donor is deferred from donation. Other diseases that can be transmitted by a blood transfusion include malaria, babesiosis, cytomegalovirus (CMV), and Epstein-Barr virus (EBV).

Hepatitis

Hepatitis is an inflammation of the liver cells. There are five, possibly seven, viruses in the *Hepadnaviridae* family. The viruses are hepatitis A; B (HBV); C (HCV), also referred to as non-A non-B; and D (called delta); E; and several new ones, F and G, whose identities are being established. Hepatitis A and E are caused by contaminated food or water and unsanitary conditions and usually are not transmitted by blood. Transfusion-related hepatitis most often is caused by the B and C viruses. Hepatitis D can only infect a person already infected with hepatitis B.

Most hepatitis cases run a course of infection to recovery. Anyone who has had hepatitis B or C is deferred permanently from donating blood. The hepatitis viruses are very hardy and not destroyed by freezing or washing blood.

hepatitis B/HBV

The most serious form of hepatitis is hepatitis B (HBV), which is transmitted through contact with blood and body secretions, and by sexual intercourse. The virus is so infectious that as little as 1 picogram in a unit of blood can cause an infection through a transfusion. Patients infected with HBV usually experience liver damage and 10% become chronically infected. Chronic HBV carriers are persons who can transmit HBV and have an increased chance of developing liver cancer later in life. Seemingly healthy individuals can be carriers and transmitters of HBV.

A positive blood test result indicates that a unit of blood is contaminated with antibodies to HBV or HBV antigens. The unit, therefore, should be discarded.

Hepatitis B Virus Vaccine

Hepatitis B vaccine is available for protection against HBV. Vaccination is strongly recommended for health care workers and other persons in routine contact with the blood and body fluids of potentially HBV-positive individuals, I.V. drug users, or anyone suspected of having HBV. The HBV vaccine is also recommended for newborns.

The HBV vaccine works by stimulating the individual's immune system to produce antibodies against HBV. If exposed to the virus, the body can mount an immune response before the virus can do damage.

The HBV vaccine is given at three separate times. After the initial injection, the other ones are spaced at 1 and 6 months. A booster shot may be needed later if the individual has a low antibody titer to HBV. Titer refers to the amount of antibody in the plasma.

titer

Hepatitis B Immune Globulin

Any unvaccinated health care worker accidently exposed to the blood or body fluids of an HBV-infected individual should receive hepatitis B immune globulin (HBIG). Exposure to HBV happens by puncture from a contaminated needle or if infected blood gets into open cuts or mucosal surfaces (mouth, eyes, nose) and by contact with body fluids. HBIG should be administered as soon as possible and within 7 days from the time of exposure. Babies born of infected mothers should receive HBIG at the time of birth. HBIG is produced from the plasma of individuals who have developed antibodies against HBV.

HBIG

HIV

Potential blood donors must have their blood tested for antibodies against the human immunodeficiency virus (HIV), the virus that causes AIDS. Any individual who tests positive for HIV is permanently deferred from donating blood.

HIV is transmitted in a number of ways including I.V. drug use (when contaminated needles are shared), sexual contact (by sperm and vaginal secretions), and by other body fluids (menstrual blood or breast milk from infected mothers). Although the risk of HIV-transmission through transfusion is small, HIV contaminated blood will transmit the virus to the recipient.

Tests for HIV

ELISA

Western blot

The enzyme-linked immunosorbent assay (ELISA) is a screening test for antibodies to HIV. Whenever the ELISA is positive for HIV the blood is further tested by the Western blot, a more specific confirmatory test. When this test is positive antibodies to HIV in the blood are confirmed.

The ELISA test for antibody is not foolproof. It measures the antibodies produced in response to HIV infection, not the presence of the virus itself. The body takes time to build up an antibody titer that registers a positive test result. The time between HIV infection and the appearance of antibodies to HIV in the blood is approximately 22 days. An individual recently infected by HIV may not have sufficient antibody titers to test positive, therefore, the ELISA will be negative for HIV and the individual can transmit the virus. An individual wanting to confirm HIV negativity should be retested 6 months after having the ELISA.

In March 1996 the AABB and FDA required that all units of blood and blood components be tested for the presence of HIV by the HIV-1 antigen test (HIV-1-Ag). This test measures the presence of the p24 antigen of HIV directly rather than antibody produced in response to HIV. Researchers believe the virus may be detected in the blood before antibody levels are sufficient to test positive.

AIDS

CDC

The Centers for Disease Control and Prevention (CDC) uses standards by which an individual is considered to have AIDS. A CD4+ T lymphocyte count of 200 CD4+ T cells/μL of blood or less indicates AIDS. Clinically, AIDS is defined by the presence of any of the following: pulmonary tuberculosis, two episodes of bacterial pneumonia, and, in women, invasive cervical cancer.

AIDS is a disease that requires the presence of HIV and other criteria be met: a low T cell count and any of the above conditions. The classic symptoms of AIDS are infections and tumors such as Kaposi's sarcoma, a purplish skin lesion; *Pneumocystis carinii* pneumonia, which is caused by a protozoal microorganism and found in individuals with a defective immune system; thrush, a fungal infection; lymphadenopathy (enlarged lymph nodes); and many more. These diseases arise because the individual's immune system cannot generate an immune response. The infections associated with AIDS are typically opportunistic infections, so called because they appear in individuals with severely weakened immune systems and not in those with healthy immune systems.

opportunistic infections

When any of the symptoms of an infection develop in an HIV-positive patient, he or she is considered to have AIDS. Individuals can live with HIV and AIDS for years, but ultimately most succumb to infections.

Individuals with AIDS lack the major components of the immune system. HIV attacks and destroys CD4+ T lymphocytes and the macrophages. The body cannot conquer any disease without these immune cells: they are essential to the communication lines in the immune response. When HIV destroys CD4+ T cells, antigen

CD4+ T lymphocytes
macrophages

Figure 15.1 HIV REPLICATION

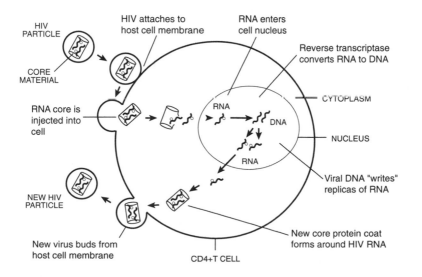

HIV attaches to host cell membrane

RNA enters cell nucleus

HIV PARTICLE

Reverse transcriptase converts RNA to DNA

CORE MATERIAL

CYTOPLASM

RNA core is injected into cell

RNA

DNA

NUCLEUS

RNA

Viral DNA "writes" replicas of RNA

NEW HIV PARTICLE

New core protein coat forms around HIV RNA

New virus buds from host cell membrane

CD4+T CELL

recognition and antibody production cannot take place. CD4+ T cells can no longer alert the phagocytes, B cells, and other immune cells to mount an immune response. In the person with AIDS, cell communication lines in the immune response are destroyed by HIV and the person succumbs to disease.

At the present time there is no cure for AIDS. Some drugs can prolong the onset of AIDS, but there are side effects. Treatment can cause chronic problems such as anemia, thrombocytopenia, and many other blood disorders. Drugs on the market and in clinical trials attempt to make the disease at least manageable.

Other Transfusion–Transmissible Diseases

The human T cell lymphotropic viruses are known to cause disease in blood transfusion recipients. They are associated with leukemia and other diseases.

CMV   Cytomegalovirus (CMV) is a member of the herpes family of viruses with the ability to infect many different types of cells, such as kidney, liver, lung, leukocyte, and epithelial. A cytomegalovirus infection within healthy adults is generally uneventful and symptoms may include a mild, mononucleosislike syndrome.

Cytomegalovirus is a problem only for individuals with an incompetent immune system. Immunoincompetent patients include bone marrow transplant recipients and patients on high-dose chemotherapy or with immune deficiency diseases. For individuals with a competent immune system, cytomegalovirus presents few problems.

Questions

Transfusion and Disease Transmission

1. True or false: The transmission of disease by transfusion has been greatly reduced but nonetheless remains a threat to transfusion recipients.

2. What role do the American Association of Blood Banks and the Food and Drug Administration have in the testing of blood and blood components?

3. Cite three diseases for which blood is tested.

4. What is the most serious form of hepatitis and how is it transmitted?

5. True or false: A seemingly healthy individual can be a chronic carrier and transmitter of HBV.

6. How can an individual be protected against contracting HBV and what individuals especially require protection?

7. How can an individual who is exposed to HBV-contaminated blood be protected against the virus?

8. True or false: As long as an HIV-positive individual is receiving medical treatment, he or she may donate blood.

9. Name three tests available for determining whether an individual has HIV.

10. Explain why an individual may test negative for HIV according to the ELISA but still be a carrier of the virus.

11. Briefly, how is the immune system affected by HIV?

12. Correct this statement: Cytomegalovirus is a transfusion-transmissible disease that can affect an individual who is immunocompetent.

16 Component Therapy

Component therapy refers to the use of a specific blood component to treat certain conditions or diseases such as anemia, leukemia, thrombocytopenia, and hemophilia. Blood component therapy has radically changed the way blood is utilized. In the early days of transfusion medicine, whole blood was given to patients who needed blood for any reason. Today, whole blood is rarely administered to a patient and then only when blood loss is significant. Aside from being unhealthy, a transfusion of a unit of whole blood when it is not needed is wasteful. A unit of whole blood administered to any normovolemic patient overloads the vascular system, posing serious problems such as edema. Normovolemia refers to normal circulating blood volume.

normovolemia

Whole blood is collected and usually processed into various components for use in component therapy. Packed red cells, platelets, and plasma then become available for many patients. For example, anemic patients (those with a low red cell count) need only red cells, not whole blood. A transfusion of packed red cells properly treats their condition.

whole blood
packed red cells
platelets
plasma

Component therapy is used when no other therapeutic modality is available to meet the current needs of the patient. The component of choice is the one that best remediates the patient's medical condition.

Cellular blood components are prepared by blood banks while pharmaceutical companies prepare plasma components as purified concentrations of plasma proteins. The latter include coagulation factor concentrates, albumin and plasma protein fraction, immune serum globulin, and growth factors.

Whole Blood in Therapy

A unit of whole blood has a volume of 450 mL and is composed of red cells, white cells, platelets, and plasma.

An anticoagulant/preservative, 63 mL, is added to units of whole blood. The Hct of whole blood is usually between 0.36 and 0.44. Whole blood is usually processed into its components.

If a patient has massive blood loss, usually greater than 25% of the total blood volume, a unit of whole blood may be given. An infusion of whole blood improves the patient's ability to transport oxygen (red cells) to the tissues as well as increasing the circulating blood volume (plasma). An infusion of a unit of whole blood raises the Hct (number of red cells) of a patient by about 0.03. Whole blood increases the ability of patients to transport oxygen by raising the Hgb concentration by about 1 g/dL.

Apheresis

Apheresis is the removal of a specific blood component or components from the circulation of a patient or donor. The removal of red cells and white cells is referred to as cytapheresis, or hemapheresis; plasma removal as plasmapheresis; and platelet removal as plateletpheresis. Apheresis is also used to remove hematopoietic stem cells from the circulation following the administration of recombinant growth factors. After high dose chemotherapy the stem cells are reinfused to stimulate blood cell production. Single-donor apheresis refers to the collection from one donor. When multiple donors contribute to a collection component, the process is simply referred to as apheresis. Single-donor apheresis is safer for the patient as risks of a transfusion reaction and disease transmission are reduced.

cytapheresis
plasmapheresis
plateletpheresis

single-donor apheresis

A specific blood component may be used to treat disease. For example, HLA-matched platelets are given to people who have received multiple transfusions and have built up numerous antibodies to HLA antigens. They are sensitized to HLA and matched platelets reduce the possibility of a reaction. The platelet reaction to HLA is loss of platelet function. HLA stands for the human leukocyte antigen and is a molecule found on most human cells including platelets. Except in identical twins, HLA molecules are genetically different among human beings.

therapeutic apheresis

Apheresis is also used to eliminate a specific problematic component from a patient's blood in a process called therapeutic apheresis. Depending on the condition, the component may or may not be replaced with an equivalent donor component. For example, in certain leukemias in which the white cell count is very high, some of the white cells are removed from the circulation to reduce blood viscosity. They are not replaced with allogeneic cells. Diseased plasma may be removed from the circulation by plasmapheresis and usually replaced with albumin.

cell separator

centrifugation

In apheresis, blood is collected by a machine called a cell separator. A sterile disposable tubing set in the cell separator collects the blood. I.V. line(s) from the tubing set are inserted into one or two veins of the donor or patient. Blood is drawn into the bowl and spun by centrifugation, which separates the component from the blood for collection. The speed of the centrifuge bowl can be adjusted to isolate a specific component by its density. Unused blood components are reinfused into the donor.

The apheresis procedure may take a number of hours to collect the desired amount of the component. There are two reasons for this: the small size of the separator bowl and the need to maintain donor blood volume. The blood volume of the donor is virtually unaffected by apheresis because so little of the component is removed.

Packed Red Cells

Packed red cells are given to patients losing blood during surgery and also to patients with anemias and other conditions such as leukemia. "Packed" simply means that most of the plasma, white blood cells, and platelets have been removed from the unit of blood.

A unit of packed red cells is prepared from a unit of whole blood from which 200-250 mL of plasma have been removed. Removing plasma increases the concentration of red cells, which in turn raises the Hct of the packed red cells in the unit. Plasma can be broken down into other components, such as FFP, cryoprecipitate, and albumin.

Packed cells are collected in an anticoagulant/preservative, CPD, CP2D, or CPDA-1. Those collected in CPD and CP2D have a shelf life of 21 days and a Hct of 0.70-0.80. Packed red blood cells collected in CPDA-1 have a shelf life of 35 days. Packed cells are stored at 1-6C.

anticoagulant/ preservative

The shelf life of packed cells can be extended when supplied with 100 mL of an additive system, which is a solution that keeps red cells metabolically active. Packed red cells collected in additive systems have a shelf life of 42 days and a Hct of 0.55-0.60. The lowered Hct is due to the volume of the additive system added to the unit.

additive systems

Packed red cells must be ABO/Rh compatible. In some emergency situations, when a specific blood group is not available, this requirement may be disregarded and compatible O- cells administered. Packed cells should not be transfused for volume expansion or to improve wound healing.

Leukocyte–Poor Red Blood Cells

Patients who receive multiple transfusions are exposed to and become sensitized to many antigens on transfused cells, particularly HLA molecules on white cells. To avoid HLA sensitization, the white cells are removed from a unit a packed red cells prior to transfusion by leukocyte depletion, which can be accomplished by the washing, centrifuging, or filtering of blood. Other terms for leukocyte-poor are leukocyte-depleted and leukocyte-reduced.

White Blood Cells

Today, white cells are used in transfusion infrequently, partly because powerful antibiotics are available. White blood cells, specifically granulocytes, are only prepared for transfusion by single-donor apheresis. They are used to transfuse the following patients: those lacking the ability to fight off infections as the result of a weakened immune system, those with decreased neutrophils (neutropenia), and those not responding to antibiotics. These patients often are undergoing chemotherapy for leukemia (cancer

granulocytes

of the white cells) or bone marrow replacement therapy. Sepsis (infection) can occur in both cases.

White blood cells are stored at room temperature, 20-24C. They have a shelf life of 24 hours. The donor must be ABO/Rh compatible because white blood cell concentrates often contain significant amounts of red blood cells, which can cause a transfusion reaction.

Platelets

Platelets are transfused (1) to treat bleeding disorders due to a low platelet count (thrombocytopenia), (2) to replace abnormal platelets, or (3) platelets destroyed by conditions such as DIC and autoimmune diseases. Platelets are prepared using two methods. They are collected for transfusion from a unit of whole blood or by plateletpheresis. Both collection methods use centrifugation to separate the platelets from the other components. Apheresis platelets are administered to patients who have become sensitized to HLA on platelet membranes and as a result have developed HLA antibodies. The volume of platelets collected by plateletpheresis is equivalent to 5 or 6 units of platelets.

plateletpheresis
centrifugation

Platelets should be Rh compatible with the recipient. They do not have to be ABO compatible unless the unit contains 5 mL of red blood cells. Compatible platelets prevent sensitization to foreign antigens as well as increasing platelet life in the recipient. If only Rh+ platelets are available for an Rh- individual, Rh immune globulin should be administered to prevent sensitization, especially in women of childbearing potential.

Rh immune globulin

At times, patients have very low platelet counts and require a large volume of platelets. Heart surgery, liver surgery, chemotherapy, and DIC are examples of conditions for which platelets pooled from multiple donors often are administered. Pooled platelets, however, increase patient exposure to transmissible diseases and the formation of platelet antibodies by the patient. Platelets must be used within 4 hours after pooling.

pooled platelets

Transfused platelets usually are not successful in stopping bleeding caused by excessive platelet destruction, for example, in idiopathic thrombocytopenia purpura (ITP), untreated DIC, septicemia, or hypersplenism (when the spleen destroys too many blood cells). In ITP a platelet transfusion will not stop bleeding because donor platelets are destroyed faster than they can be replaced.

During or after a platelet transfusion it is not uncommon for patients to have fever and chills. If a transfusion reaction does occur, the transfusion should be stopped immediately. Aspirin should not be administered to treat the fever because it inhibits platelet function.

Platelets are stored at 20-24C with constant agitation to prevent clumping. At colder temperatures, platelets become inactive. Platelets have a shelf life of 5 days.

Plasma Components

Plasma that has been collected may be separated (processed) into various components: fresh frozen plasma, cryoprecipitate, coagulation factor concentrates (factors VIII and IX), albumin, plasma protein factor, and immune serum globulin. Plasma components are used for many conditions, including bleeding disorders, liver disease, burns, shock, and massive blood loss.

Fresh Frozen Plasma

Fresh frozen plasma (FFP) is used to treat clotting factor deficiencies, including multiple factor deficiency resulting from liver disease, DIC, and coagulation complications after bypass surgery. It should not be used for volume expansion.

Fresh frozen plasma is prepared from whole blood. As soon as possible after collection, plasma is separated from whole blood and quickly frozen. Plasma treated this way retains most of the activity of clotting factors V and VIII. Plasma can be stored up to 1 year at -18C. The volume of a unit of plasma is 200-250 mL.

Cryoprecipitate

fresh frozen plasma
FFP

buffy coat

factors VIII and XIII
fibrinogen

Cryoprecipitate is a concentrated solution of coagulation proteins found in the plasma and produced by thawing fresh frozen plasma (FFP). During the thawing process a white precipitate layer forms on top of the plasma. This layer contains the cryoprecipitate and is referred to as the buffy coat. To collect the cryoprecipitate, a unit of FFP is thawed at 1-6C and the buffy coat removed. Cryoprecipitate contains high concentrations of factors VIII, XIII, and fibrinogen.

Cryoprecipitate is used to treat hemophilia A, von Willebrand's disease, DIC, and congenital and acquired factor deficiencies. The component has minimal amounts of red blood cells and therefore does not need to be ABO compatible unless many units have been pooled.

fibrin glue

Cryo is also used in the preparation of fibrin glue. Fibrin glue is a substance prepared and applied topically in surgery to stop bleeding that cannot be controlled by other means. It is made by mixing cryo with bovine (cow) thrombin and calcium (Ca^{++}). The mixture is applied to the bleeding area. Fibrin glue is applied topically rather than injected. It may transmit disease.

Coagulation Factor Concentrates

factors VIII and IX

Coagulation factor concentrates are powdered (lyophilized) concentrates produced from units of pooled donor plasma. The concentrates contain large amounts of factors VIII and IX. Factor VIII concentrate is used to treat hemophilia A. Factor IX concentrate is used to treat hemophilia B (Christmas disease) and other factor deficiencies. The concentrates are prepared by heating or washing with a detergent and therefore are unlikely to transmit viral diseases.

Albumin and Plasma Protein Fraction

Albumin and plasma protein fraction (PPF) are protein solutions used to treat patients with burns, massive bleeding, or liver failure. Patients with these conditions have a protein deficiency due either to the loss of protein or a decrease of protein synthesis by the liver. Albumin and PPF may also be used with other blood products to treat rapid blood loss and replace diseased plasma.

Albumin is a naturally occurring blood protein that is part of the plasma. It is used to treat patients who have lost a large volume of blood, a condition called hypovolemia, and those with low blood protein levels.

hypovolemia

ABO testing is not required for an albumin transfusion. Albumin does not need to be infused through a blood filter because it does not contain clots or debris. During the component preparation process albumin is heated to 60C for 10 hours. It, therefore, does not transmit HIV or HBV.

Plasma protein fraction contains a higher percentage of other plasma proteins and is less pure than albumin. PPF does not transmit disease in transfusion because it is pasteurized (heated to kill organisms) during preparation.

Immune Serum Globulin

Immune serum globulin, also known as gamma globulin, is a concentrated solution of antibodies (immunoglobulins) prepared from plasma. Patients infected with an organism too powerful for their immune system to destroy may receive plasma from a donor who has been exposed to or had the same infection. Serum containing donor antibodies is transfused or injected into the patient to provide antibodies already formed against the antigen. Immunity provided from sources outside the body is called passive immunity. Immune serum globulin is also given to patients deficient in gamma globulin, a condition called hypogammaglobulinemia.

gamma globulin

passive immunity

hypogammaglobulinemia

Recombinant Growth Factors

Recombinant growth factors are prepared by pharmaceutical companies. They are used in therapy to increase the numbers of certain blood cells. Growth factors currently used are erythropoietin (EPO), granulocyte colony-stimulating factor (G-CSF), and granulocyte-macrophage colony-stimulating factor (GM-CSF).

Erythropoietin

EPO   Erythropoietin (EPO) is a naturally occurring protein hormone produced and released by the kidney cells. A small percentage of EPO is synthesized in the liver. It stimulates stem cells to develop into red blood cells. Blood low in oxygen passing through the kidneys stimulates the release of EPO. Patients with poor kidney function are often anemic because they are unable to produce this hormone.

recombinant technology   Recombinant technology (genetic engineering) has produced synthetic EPO. A promising therapy, recombinant erythropoietin does in fact stimulate the stem cells to make red blood cells. It takes about 2 weeks before red blood cell production increases and 2-3 months for the Hct to reach the desired level. Although there may be complaints of headache and joint pain, EPO causes few side effects in the patient. Blood pressure may increase slightly following therapy, but this usually is due to the increased Hct. Erythropoietin may be administered either intravenously (I.V.) or subcutaneously (s.c.).

Recombinant EPO is used for patients with anemia due to end-stage renal disease. It is currently being applied in other types of anemia, such as in individuals with AIDS and some malignancies. Before the use of recombinant erythropoietin, patients with kidney disease and anemias were given packed red cells to maintain a normal Hct. Recombinant EPO has almost eliminated the need for blood transfusions for these patients.

G-CSF and GM-CSF

Recombinant G-CSF and GM-CSF are used therapeutically in the following situations: after a bone marrow transplant to enhance engraftment of white blood cells, after intensive chemotherapy to increase the number of white blood cells, and prior to the collection of peripheral blood stem cells (found in the circulation rather than marrow) to increase the number of these stem cells.

G-CSF is a protein with an important role in therapy. It stimulates stem cells to differentiate into neutrophils, the white cells that are the body's main defense against bacterial infections. The use of G-CSF improves the production of neutrophils and helps control bacterial infections. The drug stimulates only neutrophils. In patients undergoing intensive chemotherapy and bone marrow transplant, bacterial infections are a major cause of mortality.

neutrophils

G-CSF may be administered either intravenously or subcutaneously. Recombinant G-CSF should be diluted with dextrose in water; it should not be diluted with saline. The chief complaint, or adverse effect, of G-CSF is bone pain. Individuals receiving G-CSF may experience anemia and thrombocytopenia. Leukocytosis (an increased white cell count) may occur following therapy.

Recombinant GM-CSF is a glycoprotein used to increase the number of granulocytes and macrophages in patients undergoing bone marrow transplant or receiving high-dose chemotherapy. The drug may be administered either I.V. or s.c. Side effects from GM-CSF include diarrhea, rash, malaise or feeling of tiredness, fever, headaches, chills, and others.

CHART 5: BLOOD COMPONENTS

PRODUCT	WHOLE BLOOD	PACKED RBCS	PACKED RBCS	PLATELETS	GRANULOCYTES	FRESH FROZEN PLASMA (FFP)
AC/p	CPD, CP2D, CPDA-1	CPD, CP2D, CPDA-1	CPD - PREFERRED ADDITIVE SYSTEM	CPD, CPDA-1	CPD, CPDA-1	CPD, CPDA-1
HCT OF PRODUCT	0.36-0.44	0.80	0.55-0.60	—	—	—
VOLUME OF UNIT	500 mL	250 mL	300-350 mL	50-70 mL	200-400 mL with platelets; 100-200 mL in unit if no platelets in units	—
DISEASE TRANSMISSION	Yes	Yes	Yes	Yes	Yes	Yes, not CMV
ABO/Rh COMPATIBILITY	ABO and Rh	ABO and Rh	ABO and Rh	Rh compatibility necessary; ABO compatibility preferred, not necessary	ABO and Rh	ABO
USES IN TREATMENT	Rarely used; may be used for massive blood loss or severe burns	Red cell replacement; often used with crystalloids to increase Hct and volume	Red cell replacement; often used with crystalloids to increase Hct and volume	To increase platelet count	For individuals with low white cell count or unresponsive to antibiotics	To increase clotting factor levels; valuable in treating factor deficiencies when concentrates not available
INCIDENTALS	Rh- blood may be given to Rh+ individuals; presence of white cells and platelets may cause sensitization; should be filtered. Storage: 21 days in CPD or CP2D, 35 in CPDA-1	2 times the Hct of unit of whole blood; should be filtered. Storage: 21 days in CPD or CP2D, 35 in CPDA-1	Additive systems increase storage time to 42 day; should be filtered	Rh- patients may need Rh+ platelets and possibly Rh immune globulin. Multiple platelet transfusions may sensitize patients to HLA antigens, requiring HLA-matched platelets. Blood filter (170µ). Storage: 20-24C Shelf life: 5 days	Not accepted by Food and Drug Administration (FDA). HLA complications possible with transfusions. Storage: 20-24C. Shelf life: 24 hrs	Often used after bypass surgery. Storage: -18C Shelf life: 1 yr

CHART 5: BLOOD COMPONENTS *contin.*

PRODUCT	CRYOPRE-CIPITATE	COAGULATION FACTOR CONCEN-TRATE; FACTOR VIII	FACTOR IX	COLLOID SOLUTIONS ALBUMIN	PLASMA PROTEIN FRACTION (PPF)	IMMUNE SERUM GLOBULIN
AC/P	—	—	—	—	—	—
HCT OF PRODUCT	—	—	—	—	—	—
VOLUME OF UNIT	10–20 mL	Amount of FVIII in mgs varies by manufacturer	Amount of FIX in mgs varies by manufacturer	200 and 500 mL 5%; 50 and 100 mL 25%	5% protein solution	Varies by manufacturer
DISEASE TRANSMISSION	Yes	No; reduced risk	No; reduced risk	No	No	Yes, some, but not AIDS
ABO/Rh COMPATIBILITY	Preferred, but not necessary	Plasma compatible, but not necessary	Plasma compatible, but not necessary	No	No	—
USES IN TREATMENT	To increase levels of factors VIII, XIII, fibrinogen, and von Willebrand's factor	For treatment of FVIII deficiency (Hemophilia A)	Hemophilia B (Christmas disease)	Volume expansion when crystalloids inadequate (shocks, burns, liver failure, hemorrhage); used in severe liver disease	Used for hemorrhagic and hypovolemic shock, burns, plasma replacement during plasmapheresis	Provides immune protection; used to treat patients with low levels of gamma globulin
INCIDENTALS	Does not need to be pooled; 0.9% normal saline may be needed to assist transfusion	Lyophilized plasma derivative; obtained by fractionation; allergic reactions reduced over cyro	Also has factors II, VII, X; prepared from large pools of donor plasma; contains Vit-K dependent coagulation factors for treating warfarin overdose in certain patients	5% solution equivalent to plasma; 25% is 5 times the protein concentration of plasma		INCIDENTALS Concentrated solution of gamma globulin; prepared from pools of random donors; prepared from donors with large amounts of antibody; extracted from patients exposed to certain viral and bacterial diseases

Questions

Component Therapy

1.   Explain how whole blood is utilitized in component therapy.

2.   True or false: Whole blood is only administered when blood loss is significant, usually greater than 25% of total blood volume.

3.   What is the volume of a unit of whole blood? The Hct?

4.   Define apheresis, citing two kinds and the component associated with each.

5.   What patients are given HLA-matched platelets and why?

6.   How and why may white cells be removed from persons with certain leukemias?

7.   What is the name of the machine that collects a blood component and what is done with the components that are not isolated for use?

8.   Explain how the Hct is affected when plasma is removed from blood.

9.   Packed red cells are collected in an anticoagulant/preservative. Name two.

10.   A solution is added to packed red cells. What is the solution called and explain the reason it is added.

11.   True or false: Packed cells should be ABO/Rh compatible.

12.   a. What patients receive packed red cells? b. Leukocyte-poor red blood cells?

13.   Antibiotics have reduced the need for white blood cell transfusions. At times granulocytes are still transfused. Give two examples of patients who may require a transfusion of granulocytes.

14. Why is an adequate circulating blood volume important to maintaining life?

15. Platelets should be Rh compatible. Why is it preferable that they also be ABO compatible?

16. In an emergency, Rh+ platelets can be an administered to an Rh- individual, but what measure should be taken to ensure that the patient does not become sensitized to the Rh antigen?

17. The use of pooled platelets presents problems. Describe one.

18. What are two times when transfused platelets do not stop bleeding?

19. Name three components that may be derived from plasma.

20. What two clotting factors remain viable in fresh frozen plasma (FFP)?

21. Define cryoprecipitate and give one use for it.

22. What is immune serum globulin? Another name for it?

23. Three recombinant growth factors are used in therapy to increase blood cell production. What are their names and acronyms?

24. How long does it take for red cell production to increase and the Hct to reach the desired level in a patient who has received EPO?

25. Why is G-CSF used in patients undergoing extensive chemotherapy or bone marrow transplant?

Synthetic volume expanders are commercially prepared solutions that are used to replace lost blood volume and plasma fluid. They are normal saline, lactated Ringer's, dextran, and hespan. When added to the vascular space, synthetic volume expanders increase the volume of blood circulating throughout the body. An adequate circulating blood volume is critical for maintaining life: the flow of blood to organs depends on blood volume. If blood volume is inadequate, many organ systems, especially the heart, brain, and kidneys, do not function properly.

blood volume
plasma fluid

There are two types of volume expanders: crystalloids and colloids. Each is used to treat blood loss. Both are administered I.V. They may be used interchangeably for treating volume replacement. The medical team determines what fluid to use in a given situation.

Crystalloids

The crystalloids include normal saline, lactated Ringer's, dextrose, and various combinations of these. They often are used to replace blood loss, provide fluid for dehydrated patients, and allow direct access to the vascular system for emergency drug administration. Normal saline and lactated Ringer's are simple solutions made up of anions (negative ions, e.g., CL^-, HCO_3^-) and cations (positive ions, e.g., Na^+, Mg^{++}, Ca^{++}, etc.). Dextrose is a liquid solution of the simple sugar glucose.

Crystalloids expand the vascular space, but only for a short time because they tend to diffuse into the interstitial space or are filtered out by the kidneys. They may be used when rapid volume expansion is required.

Normal Saline

Normal saline (NS) is a naturally occurring salt solution found in the body. It is the only electrolyte solution that can be transfused along with blood or blood components.

Often infused with blood or blood components, normal saline decreases blood viscosity and does not hemolyze red cell.

Lactated Ringer's

Lactated Ringer's is often used as a volume expander. It is similar to saline, except that it contains Ca^{++}, which may stimulate clotting.

Dextrose

Dextrose is a simple sugar solution that often is administered I.V. to patients. It is never used in blood transfusion because it causes red cells to hemolyze.

Colloids

Colloids are volume expanders made up of long-chain polysaccharide (sugar and starch) molecules. Due to their molecular size and chemistry, they tend to stay within the vascular system longer than the crystalloids and are very useful in maintaining blood volume. They are used to treat certain patients, including burn patients and those in shock from bleeding, both of whom are likely to be plasma deficient. The colloids include such manufactured substances as dextran and hetastarch (also known as hydroxyethyl starch or hespan).

Questions

Synthetic Volume Expanders

1. Why are synthetic volume expanders given to patients?

2. What happens when organs do not have adequate blood volume?

3. Name two kinds of synthetic volume expanders and explain why each is used.

4. When are crystalloids used and why?

5. Why is normal saline infused with blood or blood components?

6. Provide the correct version of this statement: Lactated Ringer's must be infused with blood because it contains calcium, which is necessary to stimulate clotting.

7. What is the main difference between crystalloids and colloids?

8. What natural blood component do colloids resemble, and why, therefore, are they useful in treatment?

9. Give two examples of situations in which colloids are administered.

18 | The Uses of Autologous Blood

Autologous blood is the best possible blood for an individual to receive during a surgical procedure because there is no chance of disease transmission or a transfusion reaction. The use of autologous blood also decreases the demand for allogeneic blood. The reinfusion of one's own blood is referred to as autotransfusion. Collection of the patient's own blood or blood components for transfusion is called autologous blood recovery.

autotransfusion

autologous blood recovery

Autologous blood recovery is an underutilized method of blood replacement. Various facilities such as hospitals offer autologous blood recovery programs.

There are four autologous blood recovery methods currently available that allow patients to receive their own blood during or after surgery: (1) predonation, (2) hemodilution (3) intraoperative blood salvage, and (4) postoperative wound drainage collection.

Predonation

Predonation is used in surgical procedures during which the surgeon expects significant blood loss. Cardiac, vascular, urologic, and orthopedic operations make use of predonated blood.

To predonate blood the surgical patient must have a Hgb concentration of 11 g/dL and a Hct of 0.33. Predonation is not recommended if the Hgb concentration and the Hct are lower. Lower concentrations indicate anemia and predonation would only increase the donor's anemia.

Hgb of 11 g/dL
Hct of 0.33

Each week for a few weeks before surgery the patient donates a pint of blood. By the time of surgery the patient may have as many as four units of autologous blood in reserve should a transfusion be required. When autologous blood is not used to transfuse an individual during or following an operation, it must be discarded. It cannot be used for transfusing another individual.

121

Hemodilution

Hemodilution is the removal of a patient's blood prior to surgery and the replacement of the blood by an equal volume of crystalloid or colloid solution. The procedure is accomplished if the medical team expects the patient to lose a lot of blood during surgery. The solutions maintain blood volume. The crystalloid solution most often used is normal saline.

normal saline

Many types of surgery, such as cardiac and liver, involve hemodilution. A portion of the patient's blood is removed and replaced with crystalloid. The circulating blood volume remains the same but fewer red cells are in the circulation, which is a condition referred to as normovolemic anemia. After surgery the team reinfuses the patient's blood to elevate the Hct and provide platelets that may assist in blood clotting. The blood is kept at room temperature, therefore, the platelets may remain viable.

normovolemic anemia

Hemodilution is used in cardiac surgery. The heart-lung machine, which takes over heart and lung function, is a bypass pump that must be primed with crystalloid solution before surgery. When the procedure utilizing the pump begins, the solution enters the patient's vascular space and reduces the Hct to about 0.20-0.25. After surgery, the Hct may be elevated by the use of diuretics.

There are several advantages to using hemodilution during cardiac surgery. Blood that is hemodiluted is less viscous and flows more easily, which results in better blood flow to tissue capillaries. Hemodiluted blood flows more easily because a patient's temperature is cooled to about 28C. Patient exposure to transmissible diseases is reduced by hemodilution, otherwise, several units of allogeneic blood would be used to prime the heart-lung machine.

The absolute minimum that blood should be hemodiluted to is 0.15. The amount of crystalloid fluid used during bypass does not overload the circulatory system because the patient is given drugs to help diurese (make urine) a major portion of this fluid.

Intraoperative Blood Salvage

Intraoperative blood salvage is the collection and reinfusion of blood shed by the patient during surgery. This method of autologous blood recovery involves using one of two types of equipment: (1) wash devices that collect and wash (cleanse) blood before reinfusion and (2) nonwash devices that collect and reinfuse blood to the patient without washing. The wash device is referred to as a cell processor. The nonwash device is basically a sterile suction cannister that collects the blood shed during surgery. Blood collected by these devices is mixed with anticoagulants. CPD is used in nonwash devices and heparin or CPD in wash devices.

wash device
nonwash device

cell processor
cannister

anticoagulants:
CPD
heparin

Wash and nonwash devices are used for different surgical procedures. Neither one can be used for every surgical procedure. Both devices are contraindicated for open bowel (intestinal), bladder, and cancer surgeries or when the patient has sepsis (infection). Reinfused blood in these cases would expose the patient to possibly dangerous contaminants.

Wash devices are used in surgeries such as cardiac, liver transplant, orthopedic, and vascular. They are used exclusively in cardiac and liver due to the amount of debris generated, the drugs used, and, in some cases, the quantity of blood shed.

The use of wash devices eliminates most of the following from autologous blood: the anticoagulant, most activated clotting factors, fibrin split products, plasma-free Hgb, hemolyzed red cell membranes, drugs and other solutions used during surgery, and surgical debris and other contaminates. Any one of these particulates may cause complications for the patient.

During surgery the wash device collects blood in a spinning centrifuge bowl. When the bowl is full the blood is washed with 1500 mL of normal saline. Clotting factors, platelets, plasma, and white cells are removed from blood into a waste bag. The patient is reinfused only with red cells and a small amount of saline.

Figure 18.1 WASH DEVICE

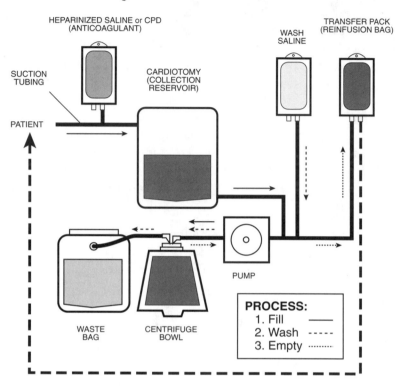

Figure 18.2 NONWASH DEVICE

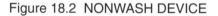

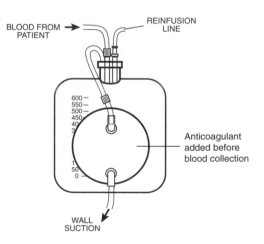

Nonwash devices do not remove surgical debris, except particulates trapped by the blood filter inserted in the I.V. line. Autologous blood reinfused by a nonwash device may contain plasma-free Hgb, debris generated during surgery, and activated clotting factors. Nonwash devices are not designed to keep up with the rapid blood loss that can occur in cardiac and liver surgery.

The decision to wash or not wash blood is up to the surgeon. Some surgeons believe that unwashed blood presents no problems to the patient.

Postoperative Wound Drainage

Wound drainage refers to the collection and reinfusion of blood that is shed postoperatively. The procedure, which has become popular recently, is a method of autologous blood recovery that helps reduce the use of allogeneic blood in transfusions given after surgery. In some surgeries – particularly total hip and knee replacements, the correction of spinal deformities, and cardiac – blood is likely to be shed postoperatively. Wound drainage devices collect and reinfuse this blood, which in the past would have been discarded and replaced by allogeneic blood. Wound drainage collection systems are smaller versions of the devices that are used to collect and reinfuse blood intraoperatively.

Questions

The Uses of Autologous Blood

1. Why is autologous blood preferred to allogeneic blood in a transfusion?

2. What are four methods of autologous blood recovery?

3. Name three operations for which the surgeon would require predonation and why.

4. True or false: A Hgb concentration of 11 g/L and an Hct of 0.33 would prevent a person from predonating blood.

5. Why does the medical team use hemodilution in cardiac surgery?

6. Describe what happens to a patient's blood in hemodilution.

7. True or false: The minimum that blood should be hemodiluted to is 0.05.

8. Explain the term intraoperative blood salvage.

9. Name the two kinds of equipment used in intraoperative blood salvage, explaining the chief difference between them.

10. What two situations – surgery and other – prohibit the use of either the wash or nonwash device?

11. Cite five contaminants that wash devices eliminate from autologous blood.

12. a. Why are wash devices used exclusively in cardiac and liver surgeries?

    b. Why are nonwash devices not used in these surgeries?

13. When a wash device is used, what portion of a patient's blood is removed? Reinfused?

14. True or false: The decision to use a wash or nonwash device is a matter of personal preference on the part of the surgeon.

15. Why does postoperative wound drainage reduce the use of allogeneic blood in transfusion after surgery?

The Concept of Blood, Page 7

1. Blood delivers oxygen, hormones, nutrients, and minerals to body cells and picks up waste products. It prevents blood loss through wound healing and is the primary carrier of immunity. Vital organs such as the kidneys, heart, and lung depend on blood for health and also process blood.

2. The formed elements are red and white blood cells and platelets. They are suspended in plasma.

3. By means of the arteries, veins, and capillaries, blood transports oxygen from the lungs and digestive products from the intestines to all body cells for use in cellular reactions and delivers deoxygenated blood to the lungs for carbon dioxide excretion

4. The average adult has 4 to 6 liters of blood.

5. Plasma is a viscous fluid that is 90% water and 10% solid matter, the latter of which includes immunoglobulins, carbohydrates, lipids, salts, vitamins, and clotting proteins.

6. Hematopoiesis is the ongoing production and regeneration of blood cells in the hematopoietic marrow. In the adult it occurs in the ribs, sternum, vertebrae, and pelvis.

7. Low oxygen in the tissues stimulates the development of the red blood cells. Infection, the white blood cells. Blood loss, the platelets.

8. The two types of marrow are hematopoietic and yellow. Hematopoietic is involved with blood cell production.

9. Red blood cells carry oxygen from the lungs to the cells. The white cells are a major part of the immune system and the platelets prevent blood loss through platelet plug formation at the site of endothelial or vascular injury.

10. Stem cells generate more stem cells and differentiate into fully mature red blood cells, white blood cells, and platelets.

11. The pluripotential cell gives rise to all blood cells.

12 Growth factors regulate the growth and differentiation of the stem cells into mature blood cells.

The Circulatory System, Page 16

1. The circulatory system is referred to as a closed loop system because blood leaves and returns to the heart.

2. Fluid and plasma components that leave the vascular system and enter the interstitial space become available to tissue cells for use in cellular reactions.

3. Blood ejected from the left ventricle enters the aorta and travels through the arteries and arterioles to the organs and tissues. Once within the capillary network of organs, blood leaves by entering the venules and veins. Blood returns to the heart by the inferior and superior venae cavae.

4. The exchange of gases, hormones, nutrients, and waste products between blood and tissues takes place at the capillary level.

5. The lymphatic system maintains the fluid/blood equilibrium of the body by returning to the circulation the fluids and substances that have left the circulation and entered the tissues.

6. Plasma proteins are too large to leave the vasculature and remain in the capillaries exerting osmotic pressure that pulls fluid back into the vascular system from the interstitial space. They are essential in helping to maintain blood volume.

7. The peripheral circulation includes the arteries, arterioles, venules, and veins outside the chest. The cardiopulmonary system refers to the blood vessels of the heart and lungs.

8. The endothelium

9. Deoxygenated blood is low in oxygen and high in carbon dioxide.

10. Deoxygenated blood returns from the organs and tissues to the right atrium by the inferior and superior venae cavae. Blood in the right atrium is pumped into the right ventricle through the tricuspid valve and from the right ventricle out through the pulmonary valve to the pulmonary arteries and lungs.

11. Oxygen and carbon dioxide

12. Oxygenated blood returns to the left atrium by the pulmonary veins. Blood is pumped from the left atrium through the mitral (bicuspid) valve to the left ventricle. From there, blood travels through the aortic valve to the aorta.

The Immune System, Page 24

1. The immune system protects the body from microorganisms and foreign substances by attacking them and rendering them harmless.

2. The white blood cells, also called leukocytes

3. Antigens are any group of microorganisms or foreign material that invades the body and illicits the immune response. The term also refers to molecules, or portions thereof, of the proteins, carbohydrates, and lipids on the surface of the invaders.

4. An antibody is a complex protein molecule produced by a mature B cell known as a plasma cell in response to a specific antigen.

5. An antigen-antibody complex is formed when an antigen is recogized by the body and the corresponding, specific antibody binds with the antigen.

6. Immunoglobulin

7. IgG is produced in greatest amounts on second exposure to antigen. IgG_1 protects the body from bacteria, except those encased in a saccharide coat. IgG_2 attacks and destroys saccharide-coated organisms. IgG_3 binds complement proteins, which enhances antigen destruction by phagocytosis. IgG_4 produces vasodilators that cause vessel pores to open. IgG_4 protects the bronchioles of the lungs and respiratory tract.

8. True

9. The cell-mediated and humoral branches. Cell-mediated responses occur when T cells recognize antigen and as a result direct immune cells to destroy antigen. T cells become cytotoxic and destroy antigen by lysis. In humoral responses, B cells mature into plasma cells to produce antibody in response to antigen. Antibody enhances phagocytosis by the macrophage.

10. Viruses attack cells from within where antibody cannot reach them.

11. Phagocytosis occurs when white blood cells engulf foreign material and render it harmless. It follows both cell-mediated and humoral responses.

12. Complement consists of proteins that assist antibodies in destroying antigen by binding to the antigen–antibody complex or directly to the antigen. Antigen complexed with antibody and/or complement is removed by phagocytosis.

13. The classical and alternative pathways. The classical pathway is activated when either IgM or IgG binds to antigens and stimulates complement activation thus enabling the macrophage to engulf the microorganism. In the alternative pathway, complement is activated by bacteria with polysaccharides on their membranes. Complement adheres to these bacteria, allowing machropages to bind and engulf them.

14. The membrane attack complex causes lysis of antigen through the action of its components.

The ABO and Rh Blood Grouping Systems, Page 30

1. ABO blood groups can be identified by the A and B antigens on the surface of red blood cell.

2. a. AB; b. A; c. B

3. Group O blood has neither the A nor B antigen.

4. Anti-A antibody and anti-B antibody are found in the plasma.

5. Anti-A antibody appears in the blood of persons in the B group and antibody-B in the A group. Both antibodies appear in group O. Neither appears in group AB.

6. Anti-A antibody agglutinates the antigens on the red cell membrane of group A blood and anti-B antibody agglutinates group B blood.

7.   Neither anti-A nor anti-B antibody agglutinates group O because this group has neither the A nor B antigens.

8.   The antigens on donor red cells agglutinate with antibodies in recipient plasma and the patient has a hemolytic transfusion reaction. Destruction of the red blood cells occurs and the recipient experiences various symptoms and even death due to the incompatiblity of donor red cells and and recipient antibodies.

9.   Group O is administered only in emergencies.

10. If an Rh- individual receives a second transfusion of Rh+ blood, antibodies developed from the first transfusion will destroy the newly transfused red cells.

11. True. Rh- blood has no Rh antigen that stimulates Rh antibody production.

12. An Rh- mother can be given Rh immune globulin.

Red Blood Cells, Page 39

1.   Erythrocytes

2.   Red blood cells are formed in the hematopoietic marrow with a life span of approximately 120 days.

3.   The main function of red blood cells is the transport of oxygen from the lungs to tissues and carbon dioxide from the tissues to the lungs.

4.   A nucleus would decrease the space available to oxygen and carbon dioxide. A nucleus would add weight to blood and increase the workload of the heart. Red cells are fully mature and do not require a nucleus.

5.   Hemoglobin, Hgb

6.   Hgb is saturated with oxygen in the lungs, and as the red cells perfuse tissue capillary beds, Hgb releases oxygen.

7.   The heme molecule attached to the α and β chains in Hgb is responsible for the red color of blood.

8.   The main function of Hgb is to transport oxygen from the lungs to the tissues. Human physiology depends on the oxygen-transport capability of blood.

9.   The three factors contributing to the optimal oxygenation of tissues are (1) blood flow to the tissues, (2) Hgb concentration, and (3) the affinity of Hgb for oxygen.

10. The three factors regulating the affinity for Hgb for oxygen are (1) the pH, (2) the PCO_2, and (3) 2,3, DPG. If one of these is not within normal limits, Hgb will not release oxygen as readily to the tissues.

11. The molecule 2,3-DPG lowers hemoglobin's affinity for oxygen so that oxygen is released to the tissues more readily.

12. Stored blood is deficient in 2,3-DPG and when patients receive large

amounts, oxygen perfusion to the tissues is minimal.

13. The shape of the red blood cell allows it to change shape when passing through the capillaries. It also provides the maximum surface area for the exchange of oxygen and carbon dioxide.

14. Polycythemia is a high red blood cell count and presents circulatory problems because the blood is so thick that it blocks the microvasculature of the lungs and kidneys. Anemia is a low red blood cell count. Not enough red cells are in the circulation to carry adequate oxygen to tissues.

15. Erythropoiesis is the production of red blood cells and is initiated by the hormone erythropoietin that is released by the kidneys.

16. Hypoxia

17. The kidneys produce erythropoietin, which is the hormone that activates the stem cells to produce red blood cells.

18. The hematocrit is the percentage of whole blood occupied by the the red blood cells. It is an index of the concentration of red cells and thus an indirect measure of the oxygen-carrying capacity of blood.

19. A Hct of 0.38 and 0.54 indicates that the number of red blood cells is within the normal range.

20. The Hct is three times the value of Hgb.

21. Hemolysis is the destruction of the red cell membrane. If large numbers of red blood cells rupture, the hemoglobin is released into the plasma. Plasma-free hemoglobin will not deliver oxygen to the tissues, therefore, the patient receives less oxygen.

22. Lungs and kidneys may fail to function if the remnants of ruptured red blood cells block the microvasculature of these organs.

White Blood Cells, p. 47

1. b. Chemotaxis

2. Neutrophils and macrophages, as well as some other white cells, destroy antigen by phagocytosis, a property by which antigen is enclosed and internalized and then destroyed by chemicals released from the cells' lysosomes.

3. Granulocytes, monocytes, and lymphocytes

4. An increased level of white blood cells indicates infection.

5. Heparin and histamine

6. If a clot forms in an infected area, the white cells cannot reach the foreign organisms to destroy them, which means the tissue will die.

7. When monocytes leave the blood they travel to the tissues where they become phagocytic macrophages.

8. Macrophages reside in tissues throughout the body where they attack

invading antigen. In the lymphatic system they function as antigen-presenting cells that introduce antigen fragments to T lymphocytes for recognition and destruction.

9. Lymphocytes recognize antigens on transplanted tissue as foreign, whereupon they produce antibodies and cytotoxic T cells that destroy the donor organ.

10. B cells are released from bone marrow and reside in the lymph nodes. When stimulated by T cells they mature into plasma cells, which produce antibody.

11. When defective T cells are not destroyed by the thymus, they recognize self tissue as foreign and destroy it.

Plasma, Page 52

1. Plasma is the liquid portion of blood in which the formed elements of blood are suspended.

2. Plasma is straw-colored, viscous, and composed of water and solutes.

3. Solutes are dissolved in the plasma and include proteins, lipids, carbohydrates, electrolytes, vitamins, and hormones. The solutes are in continuous communication with the interstitial fluid that bathes the tissue cells.

4. Interstitial fluid. It bathes the tissue cells providing nutrients for them.

5. Proteins create osmotic pressure that pulls interstitial fluid back into the blood.

6. Plasma proteins may be used by the body when the body's supply of protein is deficient. They contribute to the buffering capacity of blood, which is the body's ability to regulate the pH of blood.

7. The normal pH range is 7.35-7.45.

8. The person can experience serious health problems when pH is either too acidic or basic.

9. Normal concentrations of electrolytes are necessary for such processes as nerve conduction, blood clotting and muscle contraction.

10. c. Sodium

11. Glucose is a source of energy for all body cells.

12. Serum is plasma minus fibrinogen. If a tube of blood is allowed to stand, a clot forms on the bottom and the serum rises to the top.

Platelets, Page 54

1. Thrombocytes

2. True

3. Platelets play an essential role in hemostasis by helping to prevent blood loss.

4. Platelets go to the site of endothelial damage where they form a platelet plug.
5. Thrombocytopenia
6. Disease states can cause thrombocytopenia and thrombocytosis.
7. Nonfunctional platelets are removed by the spleen.
8. Hemostasis is the process in the body that maintains blood in the vascular system. When endothelial lining is damaged platelets form a plug and interact with coagulation proteins in coagulation.

Hemostasis, Page 60

1. They are hemostatic processes that repair injury in a vessel and inhibit blood flow from a ruptured vessel.
2. Vascular spasm is a rapid constriction of the smooth muscle fibers in small arteries and arterioles.
3. The final response is the initiation of the coagulation cascade, which leads to the formation of a fibrin clot.
4. Clot lysis must break up the fibrin clot.
5. Due to their *thick* walls... and *must* be repaired surgically.
6. Once the platelet plug has formed the platelet membrane provides a phospholipid on which activated clotting factors can bind to form a stable fibrin clot.
7. Contact, adhesion, spreading, ADP release, and aggregation
8. ADP is a chemical released by platelets that stimulates other platelets to aggregate to the site of injury
9. Prostaglandins
10. a. Thromboxane A_2 b. Prostacyclin
11. Platelet membrane phospholipids is activated when platelets are stimulated to form a platelet plug.

The Coagulation Cascade, Page 69

1. The end product of coagulation is fibrin formation of a stable fibin clot.
2. True
3. Phospholipids are needed to initiate coagulation and for two reactions within the cascade.
4. The sources of phospholipids are activated platelets and damaged tissue.
5. Fibrin would form throughout the body and coagulation factors would be consumed and not enough would be available for coagulation.
6. If any clotting factor is not available, a clot either will not form or form too slowly.
7. Calcium is essential for normal coagulation because it forms a calcium

bridge between the coagulation factors and the phospholipid, either platelet or tissue.

8. The extrinsic and intrinsic pathways

9. True

10. Current theory of coagulation states that the extrinsic pathway is the major coagulation pathway and it activates factor VII, the first factor in in vivo coagulation.

11. Factor XII is not involved in in vivo coagulation but does become activated when blood is removed from the body.

12. Vitamin K is essential for the production of clotting factors II, VII, IX, and X in the liver.

13. After a vessel has healed the clot must be dissolved by clot lysis so that blood flow can return to the vessel.

14. TPA activates plasminogen to its active form, plasmin, which breaks down the clot.

15. The D Dimer Assay evaluates the presence of FSPs in the blood.

16. FSPs are removed by Kupffer's cells, which are found in the liver and part of the mononuclear phagocytic system.

17. If FSPs were to remain in circulation, they would act as potent inhibitors of coagulation.

18. The liver synthesizes clotting factors.

19. The process of coagulation ensures hemostasis by preventing blood loss through the healing of an injured vessel.

Coagulation System Disorders, Page 75

1. False. They may cause increased clot formation.

2. Vascular integrity is the normal state of vessels that allows blood to flow through without interruption. It is lost when the vessel is damaged, surgically or by other means.

3. Loss of vascular integrity may be due to acquired (e.g., trauma) or congenital abnormalities (birth defects).

4. Defective coagulation factors mean that fibrin stabilization of the platelet plug cannot take place, therefore, bleeding occurs.

5. A congenital factor deficiency is due to a single protein abnormality, lasts a lifetime, and is rare. An acquired factor deficiency may involve multiple clotting factors, is nonhereditary, and common.

6. Both clotting and clot lysis occur in DIC.

7. Causes of DIC include burns, crush injuries, vasculitis, septicemia, red cell hemolysis, and others.

8. When large surfaces of denuded endothelium are exposed, platelets aggre-

gate and release phospholipids. Large amounts of coagulation factors are consumed when platelets release phospholipids that activate platelet aggregation and clot formation.

9. The blood components consumed during DIC are platelets and coagulation factors.

10. The patient with DIC must receive the blood products that are being consumed, such as platelets and coagulation factors.

11. A high concentration of FSPs causes platelets to become dysfunctional.

Platelet Disorders, Page 78

1. The quality of platelets refers to their ability to form a platelet plug.

2. Quality: the bleeding time. Quantity: the platelet count

3. a. Thrombocytopenia: a platelet count less than 150 x 10⁹/L

    b. Thrombocytosis: a platelet count greater than 450 x 10⁹/L

4. When platelet quality is poor, platelets may not be able to adhere to or aggregate at the site of endothelial damage.

5. Causes of a low platelet count include massive blood loss, radiation or chemotherapy, bone marrow tumors, and the immune response.

6. Causes of poor platelet quality include liver disease, von Willebrand's disease, storage defects, FSPs, and drugs such as aspirin, protamine, heparin, and dextran.

7. In DIC, massive consumption of platelets occurs in clotting.

8. Bone marrow disease

Blood Transfusion, Page 88

1. Blood transfusion is the infusion of blood or blood components for the treatment of various surgical and medical conditions. It may be required in the following situations: blood loss during or after surgery or trauma, hemophilia, internal bleeding, anemia, and replacement of a specific component destroyed by chemotherapy.

2. Autologous blood is one's own and allogeneic is someone else's, ie, a donor's.

3. Whole blood is a. collected in a blood bag containing an anticoagulant/preservative. b. usually processed into components, c. grouped and cross matched for compatibility, d. tested for diseases, and e. stored according to blood group and other criteria.

4. Pregnant women and persons with anemia, malaria, hepatitis, AIDS, and heart disease may not donate blood.

5. A blood donor is screened for serious diseases and medical conditions by means of extensive medical questioning and also tested for vital signs and the

Hct and Hgb.

6. A blood donor's Hgb concentration must be at least 12.5 g/dL.

7. A typical blood donation is approximately 1 pint, or 450 mL, or less than 1/10 of total blood volume.

8. CPD, CP2D, and CPDA-1 are placed in blood bags to prevent blood from clotting and provide nutrients for the presevation and maintenance of red blood cell viability. They are known as citrate anticoagulants/preservatives.

9. Citrate is an anticoagulant and prevents clotting by binding Ca^{++} that is found dissolved in the plasma.

10. Adenine helps maintain high levels of ATP, a high energy compound that enables red blood cells to provide better oxygen delivery to tissues.

11. The storage life of whole blood and packed red cells collected in CP2D and CPD is 21 days. In CPDA-1, storage life is 35 days.

12. Additive systems are commercially prepared chemical solutions containing adenine, dextrose, saline, and mannitol that are added only to packed red cells to increase their storage shelf life. About 100 mL is added to a unit within 72 hours of collection. An additive system increases the shelf life of packed red cells up to 42 days.

13. Blood components are stored and organized according to the ABO/Rh systems to ensure that the correct blood or component can be selected for a patient.

14. Stored blood develops storage lesions, which means that its components become less viable.

15. Blood grouping and cross matching must be conducted before transfusion to ensure that the the donor and recipient have compatible blood.

16. A reagant is a commercial product used to determine blood group. It is a strong concentration of anti-A or anti-B antibodies or red blood cells with known A or B antigens.

17. Front typing determines the presence or absence of the A and B antigens. Reverse typing determines anti-A or anti-B antibodies in the serum.

18. a. The serum contains anti-B antibody, which indicates group A blood.

    b. Group O, which does not agglutinate because it has no antigens, is indicated.

19. b. Cross matching determines compatibility between blood groups.

20. Blood filters trap hemolyzed red cells, cell fragments, plastic debris, and blood clots that may have formed during collection or storage.

21. The leukocyte depletion filter is used to trap white blood cells in a transfusion given to a patient who reacts to the major histocompatibility/human leukocyte antigen on the white blood cell membrane.

22.   True
23.   Normal saline reduces blood viscosity and unlike other I.V. solutions does not hemolyze red blood cells.

Transfusion Reactions, Page 96

1.   A transfusion reaction occurs following an incompatible ABO/Rh transfusion or patient sensitization to transfused white cells, platelets, or plasma proteins. Anti-A, anti-B, or Rh antibodies in recipient plasma cause donor red blood cells to hemolyze.
2.   True. The group B recipient has anti-A antibodies in the plasma, which will lyse cells with the A antigen.
3.   When the red blood cell is hemolyzed, hemoglobin is released into the plasma to become plasma-free hemoglobin.
4.   True
5.   The following symptoms can occur in a hemoytic transfusion reaction: flushing, hyperventialtion, tachycardia, sense of fright, urticaria, dyspnea, chest pressure, back pain, nausea, vomiting, cyanosis, fever, renal failure, and others.
6.   Renal failure is when the kidneys no longer function in cleansing the blood of impurities and the patient is slowly poisoned.
7.   The first step to be taken in a transfusion reaction is to stop the transfusion immediately.
8.   Acute hemolytic, anaphylactic shock, and circulatory overload

Transfusion and Disease Transmission, Page 103

1.   True
2.   The FDA and AABB require the testing of blood and blood components and set the standards for blood banking and transfusion in the United States.
3.   Blood is tested for hepatitis B and C, HIV 1/2, HTLV-I/II, and syphilis.
4.   The most serious form of hepatitis is hepatitis B, also referred to as HBV. It is transmitted by coming into contact with blood, body secretions, and sexual intercourse.
5.   True
6.   Hepatitis B vaccine is recommended for newborns and persons in routine contact with blood and body fluids of potentially HBV-positive individuals, I.V. drug users, or anyone thought to have HBV.
7.   Hepatitis B immune globulin is available and should be administered as soon as possible after exposure.
8.   False. An HIV-positive individual is permanently deferred from donating

blood.

9. The enzyme-linked immunosorbent assay (ELISA) is the initial screening test for antibodies to HIV. If the ELISA is positive the Western blot is used to confirm HIV. The FDA requires that all blood and components be tested by the HIV-I antigen test.

10. The antibody titer may not be high enough to register a positive test result.

11. HIV destroys communication among cells in the immune response. The virus attacks and destroys CD4+ T lymphocytes and the macrophages. The CD4+ T cells cannot alert other immune cells to mount an immune response. The body cannot recognize and destroy antigen.

12. Cytomegolovirus is a transfusion-transmissible disease that can affect an immunoincompetent individual.

Component Therapy, Page 116

1. Whole blood is processed into components: packed red blood cells, platelets, and plasma.

2. True

3. The volume of a unit of whole blood is 450 mL and its Hct is usually between 0.36 and 0.44.

4. Apheresis is the removal, or separation of a specific component from a patient or from a donor for use in another individual. Diseased components may be removed in a process called therapeutic apheresis, platelets are removed by plateletpheresis, and plasma is removed by plasmapheresis.

5. HLA-matched platelets are given to patients who have received multiple transfusions and built up numerous antibodies to the human leuckocyte antigen.

6. In leukemias with a high white cell count, some of the white cells are removed by apheresis to reduce viscosity.

7. A cell separator collects blood components and those not isolated are reinfused to the patient or donor.

8. When plasma is removed from blood, the Hct is raised due to the increased concentration of red blood cells.

9. Packed red cells are collected in an anticoagulant/preservative – CPD, CP2D, or CPDA-1.

10. An additive system is added to packed red cells to extend their shelf-life to 42 days. Additive systems keep red blood cells metabolically active.

11. True

12. a. Packed red cells are administered to patients loosing blood during surgery or in patients with anemia. b. Individuals who have received numerous transfusions possibly have developed the antibodies to HLA antigen on

donor cells. To prevent a febrile nonhemolytic transfusion reaction from occurring the white blood cells are removed from the unit of blood.

13. Patients with infections unresponsive to antibiotics and those with neutropenia (decreased neutrophils) may receive granulocytes.

14. Many organs such as the brain, heart, and kidneys require a normal circulating blood volume to function properly.

15. A unit of platelets may contain red blood cells that carry incompatible antigens and therefore it is preferred they be ABO compatible.

16. Rh immune globulin should be given to prevent sensitization of an Rh-individual to Rh+ blood.

17. Pooled platelets may transmit disease or cause the formation of platelet antibodies.

18. Platelets are not successful in stopping bleeding in patients with idiopathic thrombocytopenia purpura (ITP) and in patients with hypersplenism. Both conditions destroy platelets faster than they can be replaced.

19. Components that can be derived from plasma are fresh frozen plasma, cryoprecipitate, coagulation factor concentrates (factors VIII and IX), albumin, plasma protein factor, and immune serum globulin.

20. Factors V and VIII remain viable in FFP.

21. Cryoprecipitate is a concentrated solution of coagulation proteins in plasma produced by thawing fresh frozen plasma at 1-6C. It is used for some types of bleeding disorders.

22. Immune serum globulin is a concentrated solution of antibodies. It is also known as gamma globulin.

23. Recombinant growth factors include erythropoietin (EPO), granulocyte colony-stimulating factor (G-CSF), and granulocyte-macrophage colony-stimulating factor (GM-CSF).

24. Red cell production in a patient given EPO increases in about 2 weeks. It takes 2-3 months for the Hct to return to the desired level.

25. Patients undergoing chemotherapy or bone marrow transplant are highly susceptible to bacterial infections. G-CSF stimulates the production of neutrophils, the white cells that are the main defense against bacteria.

Synthetic Volume Expanders, Page 120

1. Synthetic volume expanders are given to replace lost blood volume and plasma fluid.

2. Adequate blood volume is necessary for the proper functioning of the brain, heart, kidneys, and other organ systems.

3. Crystalloids and colloids are both used to treat blood loss. Each expands the vascular space.

4. Lactated Ringer's, normal saline, dextrose, and various combinations of these are used to replace blood loss, fluid in dehydrated patients, and provide ready access to the vascular system for emergency drug administration.

5. Normal saline decreases blood viscosity and does not hemolyze cell membranes or cause clotting the way other crystalloids may.

6. Lactated Ringer's must not be administered to patients receiving blood because it contains calcium, which may stimulate clotting.

7. Crystalloids do not stay in the vascular space very long, whereas colloids remain longer.

8. Colloids resemble plasma and are effective in maintaining blood volume.

9. Colloids are given to patients with burns and in shock from bleeding. These patients may be plasma deficient.

The Uses of Autologous Blood, Page 126

1. Autologous blood is preferred because it does not transmit diseases or cause a transfusion reaction.

2. Predonation, hemodilution, intraoperative blood salvage, and postoperative wound drainage collection are methods of autologous blood recovery.

3. Cardiac, vascular, urologic, and orthopedic are operations requiring predonation because they involve significant blood loss.

4. False. These levels are acceptable. If any lower, anemia is indicated and predonation is precluded.

5. Hemodilution is used in cardiac surgery because a large amount of blood is needed to prime the pump. Hemodiluted blood is less viscous and therefore flows more easily providing better flow to tissues.

6. Prior to surgery a portion of the blood is removed and replaced with a crystalloid solution, usually normal saline. As a result, fewer red blood cells are in circulation. After surgery the patient's blood is reinfused to elevate the Hct and provide platelets thay may help clotting.

7. False. The minimum by which blood may be hemodiluted is 0.15.

8. Intraoperative blood salvage is the collection and reinfusion of blood shed by the patient during surgery.

9. Wash and nonwash devices. Wash devices wash blood before it is reinfused, whereas nonwash devices leave various debris in the blood.

10. Neither a wash nor nonwash device should be used in open bowel, cancer, or bladder surgery or when infection is present. Reinfused blood would expose the patient to dangerous contaminants.

11. Heparin, drugs, plasma-free hemoglobin, membranes from hemolyzed red cells, and surgical solutions and debris are eliminated from blood by wash devices.

12.   a. Wash devices are used in cardiac and liver surgeries because these operations generate much debris, require certain drugs, and during them much blood is shed.

b. Nonwash devices are not used because of the volume of blood loss and the debris generated.

13.   Wash devices remove clotting factors, platelets, plasma, and white cells by washing blood with 1000 mL of normal saline. Red cells and a small amount of saline are reinfused.

14.   True

15.   Blood shed postoperatively can be collected and reinfused, rather than discarded, thus the use of allogeneic blood is not required.

Glossary

A Blood Group One of four blood groups in humans based on the presence of an antigen on the surface of the red blood cell. The A antigen is on the surface. The plasma of group A blood contains anti-B-antibody. Group A blood can only receive group A or O packed cells.

AB Blood Group One of four blood groups found in humans. It is the least common group found in the U.S. population. The surface of red cells contains the A and B antigens. The plasma of AB individuals has no antibodies. Once referred to as the universal recipient because the individual could receive any blood group.

ABO Blood Group System The most important of several systems for classifying human blood. Used in blood transfusion therapy.

Acid-Base Balance Refers to the normal equilibrium between acids and bases in the body. It is maintained by buffer systems in the blood plasma and the regulating activities of the lungs and kidneys in excreting wastes, which prevents the build-up of excessive acids or bases in the blood and tissues. With a normal acid-base balance the blood is slightly alkaline, or basic.

Active Immunity A form of immunity in which the body provides its own antibodies against disease-causing antigens. It can occur naturally after an infection or artificially after vaccination.

Acquired Immune Deficiency Syndrome (AIDS) A serious, fatal condition in which the immune system is destroyed by the HIV virus and cannot respond normally to infections. AIDS sufferers often develop Kaposi's sarcoma and recurrent severe opportunistic infections such as Pneumocystis carinii pneumonia and fungal infections. It is the opportunistic infections that usually kill the person with AIDS.

Additive Systems Chemicals (dextrose, mannitol, saline, and adenine) added to packed red blood cells. They extend storage life to 42 days. No anticoagulative properties are associated with them. They are added only to packed red blood cells.

Adenosine A chemical compound that is a major building block of many biologically active compounds such as DNA, RNA, ADP, and ATP.

Adenosine Triphosphate (ATP) A compound consisting of adenosine, the sugar ribose, and three phosphate molecules. It is involved in many reactions concerning the storage and transfer of energy in cells.

Agglutination The clumping together of antigen-carrying cells or microorganisms as a result of their interaction with antibodies.

Agglutinin An antibody that causes clumping of a specific antigen; for example, the Rh antigen.

Alanine Aminotransferase (ALT) A liver enzyme whose presence can be tested for in a sample of blood. An elevated level indicates acute liver cell damage due to causes such as the hepatitis virus, cirrhosis, or cancer.

Allogeneic A term that refers to the genetic differences between individuals of the same species. Most often used to denote cells taken from a donor and transfused or transplanted into a genetically nonidentical recipient. The MHC molecules provide genetic dissimilarity. **145**

Allogeneic Blood Blood from a genetically different individual.

Alveoli Tiny saclike structures located in the lung where oxygen and carbon dioxide transfer takes place. They function in close approximation with the capillary network.

Amino Acid A chemical compound containing an amino group (NH_2) and a carboxyl group (COOH) that is the basic building block of proteins.

Anaphylactic Shock A severe and sometimes fatal hypersensitivity reaction to the injection or ingestion of a substance to which the organism has become sensitized by previous exposure. Symptoms include weakness, shortness of breath, edema, cardiac and respiratory abnormalities, hypotension, and shock. Death may occur within minutes of exposure.

Antibody A complex protein molecule produced by B cells/plasma cells in response to the presence of an antigen. It neutralizes the effect of foreign matter.

Anticoagulant/Preservative Any solution added to blood to prevent clotting and preserve red blood cell viability. At present, only CPD, CP2D, CPDA-1 and ACD are available for transfusion.

Antigen Any foreign protein, carbohydrate, or lipid found on microorganisms, foreign cells, or malignant cells that stimulate the immune response.

Antigen-Antibody Reaction The process by which the immune system recognizes an antigen and causes the production of antibodies specific to that antigen.

Antigen Presenting Cell (APC) A cell such as the macrophage or other phagocytic cell capable of internalizing antigen, break-

ing the antigen into peptide fragments, and presenting the protein fragments to CD4+ T cells. APCs are needed by CD4+ T cells to respond to protein antigen.

Aorta The major artery of the body that leaves the left ventricle and delivers oxygenated blood to the tissues of the body.

Aortic Valve The three-cusp valve that separates the aorta from the left ventricle.

Apheresis The removal of a specific component from the blood of an individual for whom the component is problematic or for use in transfusion therapy. Types of apheresis include cytapheresis, plateletpheresis, and plasmapheresis.

Arteriole A small branch of any artery that leads to the capillary network.

Autologous Blood Blood that is the patient's own blood. The term is usually used when referring to the administration of that blood in a transfusion.

Autologous Blood Transfusion The transfusion of one's own blood collected by predonation, hemodilution, intraoperative salvage, or postoperative wound drainage. The use of this blood eliminates disease transmission and transfusion reactions.

B Blood Group One of four groups of the ABO blood system. It has the B antigen on its surface and the anti-A antibody in the plasma. This group can receive either B or O group packed cells.

B Cell A lymphocyte important to the production of antibodies in the body upon stimulation by an antigen.

Babesiosis A rare sometimes fatal disease that can be transmitted through a blood transfusion. The organism that causes babesiosis is a protozoan parasite that resides inside the red blood cell.

Bacteria   Any of a large group of organisms found in soil, water, and air. Some cause disease in humans as well as other organisms. Generally classified as rod-shaped (bacillus), spherical (cocci), comma-shaped (vibrio), or spiral (spirochetes).

Basophil   A type of white blood cell. Normally about 1% of the total white blood cell count. Its main function is the release of histamine and heparin at the site of antigen invasion.

Binding   The process whereby two or more chemicals join. The binding of chemicals may activate, inhibit, or neutralize the chemical reaction.

Blood Clot   Blood that has gone from the liquid state to the solid state. Clot formation requires integration among many chemicals in the blood – Ca^{++}, phospholipids, and coagulation factors – all of which must be present for a clot to form.

Blood Coagulation   The process by which liquid blood is changed into a semi-solid mass referred to as a blood clot. Coagulation can occur in an intact vessel, but usually occurs with an injury to a vessel or when blood comes into contact with a foreign surface.

Blood Cross Matching   The mixing of the red blood cells of a donor with the serum of a potential recipient to determine whether the blood is compatible and can be used for a transfusion. Clumping occurs when incompatible blood groups are mixed; it does not occur when the same blood groups are mixed.

Blood Islands   A group of primitive cells found in the yolk sac of the embryo that are the precursors to all blood cells and the early beginnings of the vascular system.

Blood Transfusion   The infusion of blood or blood components into an individual for the treatment of a medical condition, disease, or blood loss due to surgery or trauma. Transfused blood may be either allogeneic or autologous.

Blood Grouping   A technique for determining a person's blood group. In grouping for the commonly used ABO groups, cells and serum are mixed with reagents to determine the blood group of the donor and/or recipient

Blood Volume   The amount of blood circulating throughout the body in the vascular system. Normal blood volume in the adult is about 5 liters. Maintaining blood volume is essential for organ function of the heart, brain, and kidneys.

Bone Marrow   A specialized, spongy, fibrous matrix found in the center of bones. Red marrow is involved in the production of blood cells and is called the hematopoietic marrow.

Bronchi/Bronchioles   The tubes, or airways, of the lungs that lead from the trachea, or windpipe, to the alveoli.

Capillaries   The smallest blood vessels in the body. They connect arterioles and venules. Only one cell layer thick, the walls of capillaries allow for the transfer of oxygen and nutrients to the tissues and the transfer of waste products and carbon dioxide from the tissues to the blood.

Carbohydrates   A broad class of molecules made up of carbon, hydrogen, and oxygen. Examples of carbohydrates are sugars, starches and some antigens. The most common carbohydrate is glucose.

Carbon Dioxide (CO$_2$) A colorless, odorless gas given off by the tissues to the blood, which carries CO$_2$ to the lungs where it is expired. Carbon dioxide levels in the blood regulate the breathing rate and the acid-base balance of the blood. Carbon dioxide is transported to the lungs as bicarbonate ion.

CD4+T Lymphocytes A subset of T cells that directs the immune response to foreign organisms. Also called helper T cells. HIV attacks and destroys the CD4+T cells.

CD8+T Lymphocyte Also referred to as the cytotoxic T cell. This T cell destroys virally infected cells, allogeneic cells, and tumor cells by lysing them with toxins.

Cell-Mediated Response The response brought about when a T cell recognizes a foreign invader and stimulates the B cell to produce an antibody or other T cells to lyse and destroy the invader.

Cell Separator The apparatus used in the apheresis process to separate blood components by centrifugation (high speed spinning).

Chemotaxis The movement by a cell or organism toward or away from a chemical stimulus.

Clotting Time The time required for blood to clot, usually determined by observing clot formation in a small sample of blood.

Coagulation Factor Any one of thirteen factors in the blood essential for blood to clot. Most coagulation factors are serine proteases synthesized in the liver.

Coumadin™ (Warfarin) A drug used as an anticoagulant in patients who have artificial heart valves or those prone to strokes. It blocks the action of vitamin K.

Cryoprecipitate The precipitate that is obtained from freezing plasma and then thawing it. Cryoprecipitate is the thin white layer that forms at the top of the plasma. It is very rich in factors VIII, XIII and fibrinogen. Used to make fibrin glue.

Cytomegalovirus A virus of the herpes family that can be transmitted through a blood transfusion. The virus usually only presents problems to individuals with deficient or defective immune systems.

Cytoplasm The fluid or jellylike substance within the cell membrane in which cellular organelles are suspended.

Deoxygenated Blood Blood low in oxygen returning from the body tissues to the heart for circulation through the lungs where it becomes oxygenated.

Diapedesis The movement or passage of white blood cells through the capillary pores in response to foreign organisms.

Diffusion The movement of a substance from a region of greater concentration to a region of lower concentration.

Diphosphoglycerate Commonly known as 2,3-DPG, this chemical is found in the blood bound to the hemoglobin molecule. It functions by allowing hemoglobin to release oxygen to the tissues and pickup oxygen in the lungs more easily.

Disseminated Intravascular Coagulation (DIC) A process that occurs in the body when clot formation and clot lysis happen together in a simultaneous, uncontrolled fashion. The treatment depends on the cause, but blood products such as platelets, fresh frozen plasma, and cyroprecipitate must be used to replace the components that are being consumed.

Donation Donating blood for one's own use or someone else's in the treatment of medical diseases and conditions.

Electrolyte An element or compound that when dissolved in a solution such as plasma produces ions. Electrolytes are essential for normal physiological processes. NaCl (sodium chloride), when placed in solution, separates into Na$^+$ ions and Cl$^-$ ions.

Endothelium A layer of flat cells that lines blood vessels and the heart. A tear or rupture of it will stimulate the coagulation system to form a clot.

Enzyme-Linked Immunosorbent Assay An initial screening test to determine whether or not blood has antibodies to HIV. If results are positive, further tests such as the Western blot are done to substantiate the ELISA.

Eosinophil A type of white blood cell, normally making up about 1-3% of the total white cell count. They are believed to be abundant in people with allergies and parasitic infections.

Erythrocyte A mature red blood cell that contains the molecule hemoglobin. The main function of this cell is to transport O$_2$ and CO$_2$ between the lungs and the tissues.

Erythropoiesis The process of red cell production that takes place in hematopoietic bone marrow and is controlled by the hormone erythropoietin.

Erythropoietin A hormone produced by certain cells of the kidneys in response to the reduction in the amount of oxygen reaching the tissues. It increases production of red cells.

Extramedullary Hematopoiesis The development of blood cells that occurs in organs other than bone marrow, usually the spleen or liver. In adults this condition only occurs in those with certain disease states.

Extravascular Describes the area outside the vascular system. Usually used in reference to fluid that has left the circulatory system and is in the interstitial space.

Fibrin An insoluble protein in the blood that along with platelets forms a clot. Fibrin is formed by the action of thrombin on fibrinogen, which is the inactive soluble form of fibrin.

Fibrin Glue A product manufactured by mixing cryoprecipitate, thrombin, and calcium. Used almost exclusively in surgery, it is topically applied to bleeding surfaces that cannot be controlled by other means. It has the potential of transmitting disease.

Fibrinogen (Factor I) A protein present in the plasma that is essential to the process of blood coagulation. Factor I is converted into fibrin by thrombin in the presence of calcium ions during the process of blood coagulation.

Fibrinolysis The process by which fibrin is broken down into smaller pieces called fibrin split products (FSPs) in the dissolution of a clot. This is a normal ongoing process in the body.

Filtration The movement of a substance, usually a liquid, through a semipermeable membrane that allows the fluid to pass but retains the particles suspended in the fluid.

Fresh Frozen Plasma (FFP) The liquid portion of blood that is removed and frozen immediately. It is used in the treatment of bleeding disorders such as DIC.

Gamma Globulin The fraction of serum that contains antibodies. It provides the chief defense against bacteria, viruses, and toxins.

Extracted from donor plasma and commercially processed, gamma globulin is used for passive immunization.

Globin   A protein found in the hemoglobin molecule.

Globulin   Any of a group of simple proteins found in the blood.

Graft-Versus-Host Disease (GVHD) An immune response generated in a bone marrow transplant or blood transfusion recipient. GVHD is caused by donor lymphocytes that recognize the recipient as foreign or not "self" and mount an attack against the recipient's cells. It usually occurs in individuals with defective or deficient immune systems.

Granulocyte   A type of white blood cell characterized by the presence of granules in its cytoplasm. There are three types.

H^+   The ion produced when an acid substance is placed in solutions such as water or plasma. The H^+ must be picked up by a basic solution such as HCO^-_3 in plasma.

Hematocrit (Hct)   The measure of the percentage of red blood cells as compared with the total blood volume.

Hematology   The study of blood and blood-forming tissues.

Hematopoiesis   The process by which blood cells are produced in the marrow.

Hemodilution   The decrease in the amount of blood in a patient prior to certain surgical procedures. The amount of blood withdrawn is replaced with an equal volume of I.V. crystalloid or colloid solution.

Hemoglobin (Hgb)   A complex protein found in the red cells containing the iron pigment heme. It functions by transporting O_2 and CO_2. In the high oxygen content of the lung, O_2 binds with Hgb to form oxyhemoglobin. After depositing O_2 in the tissues and combining with CO_2, it then forms carboxyhemoglobin.

Hemolysis   The breakdown of the red cell membrane and the release of hemoglobin to the plasma. It occurs normally at the end of the red cell's life cycle and abnormally in certain antigen-antibody reactions, on exposure to certain bacteria, during hemodialysis, and in other conditions.

Hemolytic Disease of the Newborn (HDN) A condition that arises during fetal life and is caused by an incompatibility between the mother's blood group and that of the fetus. The mother produces antibodies against fetal red blood cells.

Hemophilia   An inherited disease characterized by excessive bleeding. It occurs most often in males. There are two forms of the disease: A and B. In each form, one of the coagulation factors is missing or is produced at a reduced rate.

Hemorrhagic Disorder   A disorder of the coagulation system that causes inappropriate bleeding following trauma or surgery. An example is hemophilia.

Hemostasis   The cessation of bleeding, naturally through coagulation, mechanically with surgical clamps, or chemically with drugs.

Heparin   An injectable drug used to prevent blood clot formation. Although it has no anticoagulant effect on its own, heparin enhances antithrombin-III, the body's natural anticoagulant. It is produced from beef lung or pork mucosa for commercial preparation.

Hepatitis   A disease affecting the liver and caused by a virus. It is transmitted through contaminated blood or blood products. It has a mortality rate of 6-20%. The virus may remain in the blood for many years, making people carriers and unable to donate blood. Can cause serious damage to the liver.

Hepatitis B Immune Globulin (HBIG) An injectable product prepared from the plasma containing antibodies to hepatitis from an individual previously infected with the virus. HBIG should be administered within 7 days of contact with infected blood.

Hepatitis B Vaccine A vaccine specifically designed to prevent the individual from contracting hepatitis B. The vaccine is administered in three injections. Vaccination should be mandatory for individuals likely to be in contact with infected blood.

Histamine A chemical found in basophils and mast cells and released in allergic reactions and inflammatory responses. It causes vessels to dilate and decreases blood pressure.

Host-Versus-Graft Disease Refers to the immune response that arises in a recipient of an organ transplant. The recipient's (host's) lymphocytes attack the donor's cells causing organ rejection. Drugs are administered to suppress the immune response and prevent the disease from occurring.

Human Immunodeficiency Virus (HIV) This virus is responsible for the fatal disease AIDS and belongs to a class of viruses called retroviruses. This group of viruses has RNA as its genetic material; human cells have DNA. The virus contains reverse transcriptase (an enzyme) that allows the virus to convert RNA to DNA and insert it into the host cell. HIV mainly attacks the CD4+T (helper lymphocytes) and macrophages, thereby destroying major cells of the immune system.

Human Leukocyte Antigen (HLA/ MHC) A protein molecule found on the cell membrane of almost all body cells except red blood cells. HLA only functions as an antigen when transfused or transplanted into an individual other than an identical twin. HLA may be also referred to as MHC or the major histocompatibility complex molecules.

Humoral Immune Response The response in the body that causes the production of antibodies.

Hydrostatic Pressure The pressure in the capillaries that is directly related to the pressure generated by the heart as it pumps blood.

Hypervolemia An increase in the volume of circulating fluid in the vascular system.

Hypogammaglobulinemia A deficiency of gamma globulin within the blood plasma. It may be caused by a hereditary or acquired disorder. Individuals deficient in gamma globulin have a defective immune system and cannot generate an immune response through antibody production.

Hypothermia The condition in which the body temperature is below 35 degrees centigrade or 95 degrees farenheit. Occurs most often in elderly and young children on exposure to cold temperatures. Hypothermia may be used in some types of surgery to reduce the metabolic requirements of the body by lowering oxygen demand.

Hypovolemia A decrease in the volume of fluid circulating in the vascular system. When this condition occurs the patient should be treated with the appropriate fluids, whether blood, cystalloids, or colloids.

Hypoxia A condition in the body in which there is a decreased amount of oxygen in the tissues. If this continues for any length of time, erythropoietin is released from the kidneys and red blood cell production takes place. The amount of hemoglobin is thereby increased and more oxygen can be delivered to the tissues.

Immune Response The response generated by white cells, complement proteins, and antibody that leads to the destruction of antigen. Lymphocytes are the white blood cells that control the immune response.

Immune System The system of the body that protects humans from invasion by foreign organisms and cells. It produces the immune response to antigens.

Immunoglobulins Chemically complex protein molecules also known as antibodies. There are five classes released in the immune response.

Inferior Vena Cava The major vein of the body. It receives venous blood from the lower portion of the body and returns it to the right atrium of the heart.

Interstitial Space The space in the tissues of the body that separates body cells from one another.

Intravascular The term used to describe anything that is located within the circulatory system.

Leukemia A disorder of the white blood cells in which increased numbers of immature cells are produced. The disease may be treated with chemotherapy and/or bone marrow transplant. There are many types of leukemia.

Leukocyte The class of blood cells known as white blood cells, of which there are three types. All classes function in conjunction with the immune system to provide defense to the body.

Leukocyte-Poor Red Blood Cells Unit(s) of red blood cells with white blood cells removed to avoid possible sensitization to HLA. There are several ways white cells can be removed from blood.

Lymph A clear-to-cloudy fluid found in the lymphatic channels. It drains into the lymphatic channels from the interstitial space.

Lymphadenopathy The swelling of lymph nodes that can occur for many reasons. The condition is usually due to viral infections and is prevalent in AIDS and other viral diseases.

Lymphatic System A network of capillarylike vessels, ducts, nodes, and organs that helps maintain the fluid environment of the body. The lymphatic vessels have two large vessels – the thoracic duct and right lymphatic duct – that empty into veins in the upper chest and return fluid to the vascular system. Antigen is presented to T and B cells within the lymph nodes.

Lymph Node Tissue that acts as a filtering station along the lymphatic channels. Lymph nodes are found throughout the body and are most obvious in the armpits and groin.

Lymphocyte A white blood cell that normally makes up about 25% of the total white cell count, but increases in the presence of infection. There are two groups of lymphocytes: T cells and B cells.

Macrophage A large white blood cell that phagocytizes and digests foreign matter and debris that enter the body. It exposes digested antigens on its cell membrane and presents them to T cells. Some macrophages are fixed in organs such as the liver, spleen, and tissues, while others are found circulating in the blood.

Malaria A blood disease endemic to many areas of the world that can be transmitted through a blood transfusion or mosquito bite. The organism that causes malaria is a protozoan parasite that lives in the red blood cell. Infection permanently prohibits blood donation.

Megakaryocyte A cell found in the hematopoeitic marrow.Platelets originate from it by fragmentation of the cytoplasm of the megakaryocyte.

Monocyte A white blood cell that leaves the circulation and enters the tissue. Upon entering the tissue this cell matures into a macrophage.

Mononuclear Phagocytic System Aggregates of macrophages in various organs and tissues such as the liver, spleen, and lung. Also referred to as the recticuloendothelial system.

Mucus A viscous fluid secreted by mucous membranes. It acts as a protective barrier over these membranes. A lubricant that consists chiefly of glycoproteins, particularly mucin.

Neutrophil A granular white blood cell that is phagocytic and engulfs bacteria and debris. An increase in the number of neutrophils occurs during an acute infection.

Nonwash Device An autologous blood recovery system that collects whole blood shed during surgery. When the system is full, blood is filtered and reinfused to the patient. No cleansing of the blood occurs.

Nucleus A protoplasmic body in a living cell containing the hereditary material of the cell and controlling the metabolism, growth, and reproduction of the cell. Enucleated refers to the absence of a nucleus.

O Blood Group One of the four groups of blood found in the ABO system. It has no antigens on its surface and was once considered the universal donor.

Opportunistic Infection Any infection that attacks an individual with a compromised immune system, as in the disease AIDS.

Opsonization The process by which opsonin molecules produced by certain antibodies (e.g., IgM and IgG) and/or certain complement proteins bind to the surface of antigens and enhance phagocytosis.

Organ Rejection The term used to describe the immune response generated against the donor organ following transplant. Organ rejection may be generated within the recipient or be caused by donor lymphocytes in the transplanted organ.

Osmosis The movement of water against a concentration gradient.Water moves through a semipermeable membrane from a region of lower solute concentration to a region of higher solute concentration.

Oxygen (O_2) A colorless, odorless gas that is essential to all cells of the body for normal respiration and metabolism.

Oxygenated Blood Blood that has passed through the lungs and exchanged its carbon dioxide for oxygen. It is pumped from the left venuicle to the various organs and tissues of the body.

Packed Red Cells A blood component derived from whole blood by removing most of the plasma. Now the most common form of blood used in transfusion to replace lost blood or improve anemic conditions. The only component that can be stored in additive systems.

Parasite An organism that lives on or in the host deriving nourishment from it. Some parasites cause inflammation, while others cause infection and destroy tissue. Human parasites include fungi, yeast, bacteria, protozoa, worms, and viruses.

Passive Immunity Immunity that occurs when antibodies are produced from sources outside the body, such as transferring cells or serum from an immunized individual to one who is not immunized. Provided to young children to prevent the development of certain diseases, diptheria, for example.

Perfusion   The passage of fluid through the capillaries. Used in reference to blood flow through the lungs and tissues.

pH   The logarithmic term used to describe the acidity or alkalinity of a solution. It directly measures the H⁺ concentration of a solution. If the pH is low the solution is acidic; if high the solution is alkaline.

Phagocyte   A white blood cell that surrounds and engulfs foreign organisms and debris.

Phagocytosis   The process by which certain cells engulf and digest organisms. Usually performed by white blood cells in response to foreign invaders.

Phospholipids   Any of a class of compounds containing a nitrogenous base, phosphoric acid, and a fatty acid. They are found in many cells of the body and function in many important biological reactions, particularly coagulation.

Plasma   An acellular, colorless fluid that is the liquid portion of blood. It consists of water, electrolytes, glucose, fats, hormones and proteins. The formed elements of blood are suspended in this medium.

Plasma Cell   A transformed B cell that produces antibodies in response to antigen.

Plasma-Free Hemoglobin   Hemoglobin that is released from damaged red blood cells. It is released into the plasma where it is removed from the body by the kidneys. May tinge the urine a pink color.

Plasmin   The enzyme found in the blood that digests fibrin, which results in clot lysis, or dissolution.

Plasminogen   The inactive form of plasmin that circulates in the blood until cleaved into plasmin by factor XIIa or tissue plasminogen activator (TPA).

Platelet   A diskshaped, small, enucleated body found in the blood that is essential for coagulation.

Polycythemia   A serious life-threatening condition characterized by too many red blood cells in the circulation, making blood flow through the capillaries difficult. Patients often undergo therapeutic phlebotomy for removal of the excess red blood cells.

Pooled Platelets   Platelets collected from multiple donors and mixed together for use in transfusion. Multiple donors increase the chance of disease transmission and transfusion reaction. Pooled platelets are often used after bypass surgery.

Pore Size   The size of the opening in a blood filter. Filters have different pore sizes depending on their intended use. Standard blood filters in administration sets have pore sizes of 150-270 μ. They filter out large particles. Microaggregate filters have pore sizes that range from 20-40 μ and can filter out very small particles.

Predonation   Refers to the collection of autologous blood weeks before its anticipated need during surgery. The individual may donate up to four pints depending on the estimated needs of the operation.

Red Marrow   The hematopoietic marrow in the center of bones, especially the ribs, pelvis, sternum, and vertebrae. This marrow is responsible for blood cell production.

Renal Failure   Also known as kidney failure, this condition occurs when the kidneys no longer cleanse the blood. There are many causes, one of which is an incompatible transfusion reaction.

Reticuloendothelial System   A unit of the body made up of phagocytic cells: Kupffer's cells of the liver, macrophages, and cells of the spleen and bone marrow. The system functions in the immune response by fighting infection and ridding the body of cellular debris. Now more commonly called the mononuclear phagocytic system (MPS).

Retrovirus   A family of viruses with RNA as its genetic material; most organisms have DNA. HIV is a retrovirus.

Rh Antigen   An antigen present on the red blood cell of about 85% of the population. Persons having the antigen are designated as Rh positive. Blood for transfusions must be classified for Rh as well as ABO grouped.

Right Lymphatic Duct   The lymphatic duct that drains lymphatic fluid from the right side of the body and returns it to the circulatory system.

Septicemia   The widespread destruction of tissue due to the presence of bacteria or their toxins in the blood. Can be the cause of DIC.

Serine Proteases   A term synonymous with the coagulation factors. It describes the type of chemical that makes up the coagulation factors. Enzymes that cleave, or split, molecules. In coagulation, the splitting of molecules, which confers activity on them.

Serum   Plasma minus fibrinogen. If left to stand, a sample of blood forms a clot at the bottom of the tube. The remaining fluid portion is called serum.

Single-Donor Apheresis   A procedure whereby a specific component is removed from a donor's blood and used to treat a disease or condition in another individual.

Stem Cell   An immortal cell that is able to produce all the cells within the blood system.

Superior Vena Cava   The major vein of the body that drains the upper portion of the body and returns the blood to the right atrium of the heart.

T Cells   Small lymphocytes that mature in the thymus and are the chief agents in the cell mediated immune response. They stimulate B cells to produce antibodies and T cells to lyse antigen.

Thoracic Duct   One of the two major vessels of the lymphatic system that drains lymphatic fluid from the left side of the body and returns it to the circulatory system.

Thrombin   A coagulation factor found in the plasma and formed from prothrombin, factor X, and calcium. It cleaves fibrinogen to fibrin and is necessary for clotting.

Thrombocyte   A blood platelet. See Platelets, Chapter 8.

Thrombocytopenia   A condition characterized by a lower than normal platelet count. Results in bleeding and easy bruising. The causes include drug use, the immune response, neoplastic diseases, and radiation.

Thrombocytosis   An increase of platelet numbers within the blood. It is a disease state usually caused by a disease of the stem cells. The condition may cause increased bleeding or increased clot formation.

Thromboplastin   The name for the phospholipid released from damaged tissue and used in the coagulation of blood in the extrinsic pathway of coagulation.

Thrombotic Disorder An abnormality of the blood that causes increased blood clot formation within the vasculature. It may be caused by either a hereditary or acquired defect.

Tissue Plasminogen Activator (TPA) A fibrinolytic agent that causes fibrinolysis at the site of clot formation. Currently used to treat acute heart attacks due to blood clot.

Transfusion Reaction The reaction by the body to the infusion of a blood group or blood component. It may be mild or severe and in the latter lead to death. The reaction occurs when antigens or antibodies of donor blood react with antigens or antibodies in the recipient's plasma. The most serious reactions usually involve red cells that are hemolyzed upon transfusion.

Vaccine A weakened or killed disease-producing virus that is administered by injection or mouth to induce active immunity to a specific disease; for example, the polio vaccine.

Vascular Integrity The term used to describe the vessels of the body when they are intact and circulating blood in an uninterrupted fashion.

Vascular Space The term used to describe that area occupied by the vessels of the vascular system; used when referring to the blood or fluid in circulation.

Vascular System Another name for the circulatory system.

Vasculature A term used to describe the vessels of the circulatory system. Most often used in connection with the capillaries, in which case, the term microvasculature is used.

Vasculitis An inflammation in the vessels of the body. Can be caused by a number of disease states and lead to DIC.

Viremia The presence of virus or virus particles in the blood.

Virus A small protein-covered core of nucleic acid that is not considered living, but that can reproduce itself in the host cell. The protein coat is called a capsid.

Vitamin K A fat-soluble vitamin essential for blood coagulation and important in certain energy transfer reactions. It is found in green leafy vegetables, egg yoke, yogurt, and fish liver oils.

Warfarin An anticoagulant with the trade name Coumadin™. It is used to prevent blood clots from forming. It works by blocking the action of vitamin K.

Wash Devices The systems used during surgery to collect, wash, and reinfuse autologous blood. They are used in intraoperative blood salvage and in postoperative wound drainage collection. Only red blood cells and a small amount of saline are reinfused; all other components are washed into a waste bag.

Western Blot Test A more specific blood test for HIV than the ELISA. It detects the presence of antibodies to HIV in a blood sample. The test is usually done following two positive results from an ELISA. A confirmatory result is indicative of an HIV infection.

Whole Blood Blood that has had no components removed from it. It is collected in an anticoagulant/preservative: CPD, CP2D, or CPDA-1. Usually processed into its components for multiple uses.

Yellow Marrow   The nonhematopoietic marrow that is found at the ends of long bones. It consists mostly of fat.

Appendix

/	= per
g	gram; 454 grams = 1 pound
	28.350 grams = 1 ounce
mg	milligram; 1 milligram = .001 gram
µg	microgram = .000001 gram
kg	kilogram; 1 kilogram = 1,000 grams;
	2.046 pounds
mM	millimole, or .001 of a mole
	mole = 1 gram molecular weight of a substance
liter	1000 mL = 1.056 liquid quart
dL	deciliter = .1 liter
mL	milliliter = .001 liter
µ	micron = .000001 meter
mm	.001 meter = .25 inch

NORMAL BLOOD VALUES

Red Blood Cells
Females $4.2 - 5.4 \times 10^{12}/L$, or $4.2 - 5.4 \times 10^{6}/\mu L$
Males $4.6 - 6.2 \times 10^{12}/L$, or $4.6 - 6.2 \times 10^{6}/\mu L$

Hemoglobin
Females   12 - 16 g/dL, or 120 - 160g/L
Males   13.5 - 18 g/dl, or 135 - 180g/L

Hematocrit
Females   0.38 - 0.47
Males   0.40 - 0.54

Plasma-Free Hemoglobin   less than 10 mg/dL

White Blood Cells
$4.5 - 11 \times 10^{9}/L$, or $4.5 - 11 \times 10^{3}/\mu L$
    Neutrophils 60% of white cell count
    Eosinophils 3% of white cell count
    Basophils 1% of white cell count
    Lymphocytes 30% of white cell count
    Monocytes 6% of white cell count

Platelets
$150 - 450 \times 10^{9}/L$, or $150 - 450 \times 10^{3}/\mu L$

Electrolytes
> Sodium 138 - 148 mM/L
> Potassium 3.5 - 5.2 mM/L
> Calcium 8.5 - 0.5 mK/L
> Chlorine 98 - 111 mM/L

Total Blood Volume
70 ml/kg adults
90 ml/kg children

NORMAL BLOOD GAS VALUES

	Arterial	**Venous**
pH	7.35 - 7.45	7.32 - 7.42
pCO_2	35 - 45 mm	Hg 41 - 51 mm Hg
pO_2	80 - 100 mm Hg	25 - 40 mm Hg

The term mm Hg means millimeters of mercury pressure. It is the pressure exerted by blood gases in the vascular system.

BLOOD CLOTTING TIMES

Partial Thromboplastin Time (PTT) 24 - 37 seconds
Prothrombin Time (PT) 10 - 12 seconds
Thrombin Time (TT) +/- 5 second of control
Bleeding Time (BT) 9 - 12 minutes
Fibrinogen Level 150 - 350 mg%
D Dimer 3 mg/L or 3µg/mL

BLOOD TESTS TO EVALUATE COAGULATION

Partial Thromboplastin Time This test measure the intrinsic pathway of coagulation. For this test a sample of blood is removed from the patient and placed in a test tube to which platelet factor-3 has been added. The tube is gently heated and then agitated. After the reactants are mixed the timer is started. It is stopped when a fibrin clot appears. If a clot does not appear or clotting time is longer than it should be, an abnormality in the intrinsic pathway is indicated.

Prothrombin Time This test measures the extrinsic pathway of coagulation. A sample of blood is removed from the patient and placed in a test tube to which tissue thromboplastin has been added. Tissue thromboplastin stimulates the extrinsic system.) The tube is heated and agitated. After the reactants are mixed, the timer is started. It is stopped when a fibrin clot appears. If a clot does not appear or clotting time is longer than it should be, an abnormality in the extrinsic pathway is indicated.

Thrombin Time This test measures the final common pathway. It is used to determine the amount of the quality of fibrinogen in the patient's system. A sample of blood is removed from the patient and added to the test tube to which thrombin has been added. The tube is heated and then agitated. The timer is started right after the reactants are added and stopped when a clot appears. If a clot does not appear or the clot-forming time is longer than it should be, there is an inadequate amount of fibrinogen or there are fibrin split products in the sample.

Fibrinogen Determination A sample of blood is removed from the patient and added to a test tube to which an abundance of thrombin has been added. The more fibrinogen in the sample, the shorter the time before a fibrin clot appears. If the fibrinogen concentration is low or of an abnormal type, the clotting takes longer than normal.

Bleeding Time and Platelet Count The platelet count is performed by looking at a blood smear under a microscope or automated platelet counter. The number of platelets in the field of view are counted and tells the lab technician the number of platelets in the circulation.

The bleeding time test is performed right on the patient. A blood pressure cuff is placed on the upper arm and inflated to 40 mm Hg of pressure. At the same time, a scratch is made on the underside of the forearm and a timer started. The blood is blotted away every 30 seconds until bleeding has stopped. When no more blood appears the timer is stopped. Normal bleeding time occurs within 9 to 12 minutes from the beginning of the test. The bleeding time is abnormal if there is an insufficient number of platelets or the quality of platelets is poor.

D Dimer Assay This is an immunoprecipitation assay used to determine the level of fibrin split products within the blood. The sample of blood is drawn into a tube and the blood allowed to clot. The serum that remains after the clot has formed is mixed with latex (plastic) beads that contain fibrin split products attached to them. The latex beads and serum are mixed on a glass slide. If immunoprecipitation occurs, a positive reaction is noted. The normal results of this assay are less than 3 mg/L or 3 μg/mL.

Bibliography

Abbas, Abul K., M.B.B.S.: Lichtman, Andrew H., M.D., Ph.D.; Parker, Gordon S., M.D., Ph.D. *Cellular and Molecular Immunology* (Philadelphia: W.B. Saunders, 1992)

American Medical Association. *Drug Evaluations Annual 1994 (Milwaukee, WI; American Medical Association, 1994)*

Benjamin, Eli, M.D.: Leskowitz, Sidney, M.D., *Immunology: A Short Course* (New York: John Wiley & Sons, 1992)

Beutler, Ernest, M.D. senior ed., et al. *Williams Hematology, 5th ed.* (New York: McGraw-Hill, Inc., 1995)

Buck, William S., M.D. ed. *Hematology, 5th ed.* (Cambridge, MA: MIT Press, 1991)

Coltran, Ramzi, M.D. senior ed. et al. *Robbin's Pathologic Basis of Disease, 5th ed.* (Philadelphia: W.B. Saunders, 1994)

Cunningham, F. Gary, M.D. senior ed. *William's Obstetrics, 19th ed.* (Norwalk, CT.: Appleton & Lange, 1993)

De Shazi, Richard D., M.D., senior ed. *Primer on Allergic and Immunologic Disorders.* Prepared by the American Academy of Allergy and Immunology (Journal of the American Medical Association, Nov. 25, 1992, Vol. 268, No. 20)

DeVita, Vincent T., M.D.; Hellman, Samuel, M.D.; Rosenberg, Steven A., M.D., Ph.D., eds. *Cancer Principles and Practice of Oncology, 4th ed.* (Philadelphia: J.B. Lippincott Co., 1993)

DeVita, Vincent T., M.D.; Hellman, Samuel, M.D.; Rosenberg, Steven A., M.D., Ph.D., eds. *Etiology, Diagnosis, Treatment, and Prevention, 3rd ed.* (Philadelphia: J.B. Lippincott Co., 1992)

Guyton, Arthur C., M.D. *Textbook of Medical Physiology, 8th ed.* (Philadelphia: W.B. Saunders Co., 1991)

Haskell, Charles M., M.D. ed. *Cancer Treatment, 3rd ed.* (Philadelphia: W.B. Saunders, 1990)

Hathaway, William E., M.D.; Goodnight, Scott H. Jr., M.D. *Disorders of Hemostasis and Thrombosis* (New York: McGraw-Hill, 1993)

Henry, John B., M.D. *Clinical Management By Laboratory Methods, 18th ed.* (Philadelphia: W.B. Saunders, 1991)

Holland, James F., M.D.; Frei, Emil, III, M.D.; et al. *Cancer Medicine, 3rd ed.* (Philadelphia: Lea and Febinger, 1993)

Lawlor, Glen, J., M.D.; Fischer, Thomas J., M.D.; Adelman, Daniel C., M.D. *Manual of Allergy and Immunology, 3rd ed.* (Boston: Little Brown and Company, 1995)

Lee, Richard G., M.D. et al; *Wintrobe's Clinical Hematology, Vols. I, II, 9th ed.* (Philadelphia: Lea and Febinger, 1993)

Malley, William J., M.S., R.R.T., CPFT. *Clinical Blood Gases* (Philadelphia: W.B. Saunders, 1990)

Mollison, P.L., M.D.; Engelfriet, C.P., M.D.; Contreras, Marcella, M.D.; *Blood Transfusion In Clinical Medicine, 9th ed.* (London: Blackwell Scientific Publications, 1993)

Reynolds, James E.F., M.D. ed. Martindale. *The Extra Pharmacopeia, 30th ed.* (London: The Pharmaceutical Press, 1993)

Roitt, Ivan M., M.D.; *Essential Immunology, 8th ed.* (London: Blackwell Scientific Publications, 1994)

Rossi, Ennio C., M.D.; Simon, Toby L., M.D.; Moss, Gerald S., M.D. eds. *Principles of Transfusion Medicine* (Baltimore: Williams and Wilkens, 1991)

Scanlon, Craig, Ed.D., R.R.T.; *Egan's Fundamentals of Respiratory Care, 6th ed.* (St. Louis: Mosby, 1995)

Stites, Daniel P., M.D., Terr, Abba I., M.D., Parslow, Tristram G., M.D. *Basic and Clinical Immunology, 8th ed.* (Norwalk, CT: Appleton & Lange, 1994)

Valeri, C. Robert, M.D. *Physiology of Blood Transfusion* (Boston: Naval Blood Research Laboratory, Boston University School of Medicine, March 1, 1989)

Voet, Donald; Voet, Judith. *Biochemistry* (New York: John Wiley & Sons, 1990)

West, John B., M.D., Ph.D. *Respiratory Physiology, 4th ed.* (Baltimore: William and Wilkens, 1990)

Index

A blood group, 25, 145
AB blood group, 25-27, 145
ABO blood group system, 25-29, 145
  antigens and, 25
  blood groups and administered blood, 25-27, 79, 83, 84-85
  Rh antigen, 27-29, 155
  transfusion reactions, 90-91
acid-base balance, 145
acidosis, 50
acquired factor deficiencies, 71
acquired immune deficiency syndrome (AIDS), 145
  Centers for Disease Control and Prevention (CDC) standards, 100
  enzyme-linked immunoassay (ELISA) blood test, 100
  human immunodeficiency virus (HIV) and, 99-101
  symptoms of, 100-101
  and transfusions, 80, 81, 97, 99
  Western blot blood test, 100
active immunity, 145
additive systems 82-83, 107,145
adenine, 82, 83
adenosine, 145
adenosine triphosphate (ATP), 82, 145
agglutination, 25, 84-85, 145
agglutinin, 145
AIDS. See acquired immune deficiency syndrome (AIDS)
albumin
  component therapy, 115
  and plasma protein fraction (PPF), 110-111
allergies and IgE antibody, 18-19, 43
allogeneic, 145
  blood, 25, 79, 146
  cells, 20
ALT (alanine aminotransferase), 97, 145
alternative pathway, 23
alveolar-capillary network, 14
alveoli, 14-15, 146
American Association of Blood Banks (AABB), 83, 97
amino acid, 146
anaphylactic shock, 94, 146

anemia, 35, 79, 112
antibodies (Abs), 17-23, 146
  anti-A and anti-B, in blood groups, 25, 84-85
  classes of, 18
  complement system, 21-23
  production of, 45, 46
  Rh antigen, 27-29
  transfusion reactions, 90
anticoagulants, 146
  Coumadin™. See also heparin. (Warfarin), 67
  donated blood, 79-82
  interoperative blood salvage, 123
  preservatives, 81-82, 146
antigen-presenting cell (APC), 44, 46, 146
antigens (Ags), 12, 17-23, 41, 146
  A and B, in blood groups, 25, 84-85
  antigen-antibody complex, 18-19
  antigen-antibody reaction, 146
  human leukocyte antigens (HLA/MHC), 85, 105, 107, 151
  lymph nodes, 12
  markers, 81
  transfusion reactions, 90
  white blood cells, 41-46
aorta, 8, 13,14, 146
aortic valve, 14, 146
apheresis, 105-106, 146
arteries, 8, 13, 55, 57
arteriolar end, 10, 12
arterioles, 8, 13, 55, 146
artherosclerosis, 71
aspirin therapy, 58
autoimmune diseases, 46
autoimmunity, 46
autologous blood, 79, 146
  autotransfusion, 121
  hemodilution, 122
  intraoperative blood salvage, 123-135
  postoperative wound drainage, 125
  predonation, 121, 154
  recovery methods, 121-125
  transfusion, 146. See also transfusion

B blood group, 25, 146
B cells, 18, 20, 42, 45-46, 146

babesiosis, 97, 146-147
bacteria, 147
banked (stored) blood
  and 2,3-DPG, 34
  additive systems, 82-83
  anticoagulants in, 81-82
  blood bank system, 83
  blood donations, 79-81
  citrate anticoagulants/preservatives (CPD, CP2D, CPDA-1), 81-82, 107, 123
  coagulation factors and, 61, 83
  defects in, 83-84
  donor health, 79-80
  filters, 85-87
  shelf life, 82
  storage lesion, 83
  storage system, 83
  testing, 81, 97
basophils, 42, 44, 147
bicuspid valve, 15
binding, 147
bleeding and coagulation factor disorders, 71-74
bleeding time test, 76
blood
  administration, 86-87
  allogeneic, 25, 79, 145
  autologous, 79, 121, 146
  banks, 83
  circulation. See circulatory system
  clot, 147
  compatibility, 25-29, 84-85, 90-91
  components 81, 82, 83, (table) 114-115
  cross matching, 79, 84-85, 147
  donations, 79-81, 97-102
  filtering, 85-86
  function and components, 1-2, 79
  grouping, 79, 83, 84-85, 147. See also ABO blood grouping
  islands, 3, 147
  origin of, 2-3
  pH, 48
  plasma, 1, 25, 48-51
  stored. See banked (stored blood)
  volume, 1-2, 12, 48, 118, 121, 147
blood cells, 1-2. See also red blood cells; white blood cells; platelets
  committed, 6
  conditions stimulating production, 2-3
  differentiation, 6

growth factors, 6, 111-113
life span, 5
origin of, 2-3
production in bone marrow, 3, 5, 37. See also bone marrow
production in fetus, child, and adult, 3
stem cells, 6
types of, 5
blood filters, 85-87
blood islands and fetal growth, 3
bone marrow, 2, 3, 5, 147
  blood cells, released from, 31
  composition of, 3, 5
  diseases, 77
  red (hematopoietic), 3, 5, 6, 154
  stem cells production, 2-3, 6, 37
  transplants, 5, 6, 108, 112
  yellow, 3, 5, 157
buffering, 48
buffy coat, 110
bronchi/bronchioles, 43, 147

calcium in blood, 50, 62, 82
cancer and cell-mediated responses, 20
capillaries and capillary bed, 8, 10, 147
  in peripheral circulation, 13
  in cardiopulmonary system, 13-15
capillary pores, 10, 48
  diapedesis of, 41
carbohydrates, 147
carbon dioxide, 14, 31, 148
cardiopulmonary system, 13-15
CDD4+ T lymphocytes, 101-102
CD8+ T lymphocytes, 148
cell lysis, 45
cell-mediated immunity, 19-21, 46
cell-mediated response, 19-21, 148
cell processor wash system, 123
cell separator, 106, 148
cellular differentiation, 6
cellular metabolism, 1, 84
centrifugation, 106
cerebral vascular accident (CVA), 58
chemotaxis, 41, 148
chemotherapy, 5, 6, 76-77, 79, 102, 107
chlorine in plasma, 50
circulatory overload, 94
circulatory system, 1, 8-10
  oxygen transfer from blood, 31-34
citrate anticoagulants/preservatives (CPD,

CP2D, CPDA-1), 81-82, 107, 123
classical pathway, complement, 22-23
clot lysis, 55, 68
clotting, 2, 44
    aspirin therapy to reduce, 58
    factors, 57, 61-67, 109-110
    mechanism of, 61-67
    platelets, aid in, 5, 53, 55-59
    thrombocytosis and, 77
clumping, 25, 109. *See also* agglutination
coagulation. *See also* clotting
    activation, 62
    anticoagulants, 67, 81-82
    blood tests to evaluate, 71
    cascade, 22, 55, 61-68
    clot lysis, 55, 68
    disorders, 64, 71-74
    factor concentrates, 110, 115
    factors, 51, 61-67, 71-74, 148
    fibrin split products (FSPs), 68
    final common pathway, 65
    in vitro, 64
    in vivo, 64, 65-67
    pathways, 64-67
    platelets and, 53
    phospholipids, 62
    vitamin K and Coumadin ™, 67
colloids, 115, 118-119
committed blood cells, 6
compatibility, ABO blood grouping, 25-29,
    84-85, 90-91
complement proteins, 17, 19, 21-23
complement system, 21-23. *See also* immune
        system
    antigens and, 21
    and foreign surfaces, 21
    hemolysis, 21
    IgM and IgG antibodies, 18, 19, 22-23
    pathways, 22-23
    and phagocytosis, 21
    protein activation, 22
    vascular permeability, 21
    and white blood cells, 43
component therapy, 104-115
    albumin and plasma protein fractions
        (PPF), 110-111
    apheresis, 105-106
    blood components (table), 114-115
    coagulation factor concentrates, 110
    cryoprecipitate, 110

erythropoietin (EPO), 112
fresh frozen plasma (FFP), 65, 73, 109,
    110, 114, 149
G-CSF and GM-CSF, 112-113
immune serum globulin, 111
leukocyte-poor (-depleted) red blood cells,
    107, 152
packed red cells, 106-107
plasma components, 109-111
platelets, 108-109
recombinant growth factors, 111-112
white blood cells, 107-108
whole blood, 104-105
congenital factor deficiency, 71
Coumadin™ (warfarin), 67, 148
CPD, CP2D, and CPDA-1, 81-82, 107, 123
cross matching, 25-27, 84-85
cryoprecipitate, 73-74, 110, 115, 118
crystalloids, 118-119, 122
cyclosporine, 45
cytapheresis, 105
cytomegalovirus (CMV), 97, 102, 148
cytotoxic T cells, 19, 46, 148
cytoplasm, 44, 53, 148

D antigen. *See also* Rh
deoxygenated blood, 14, 148
dextrose, 81-82, 83, 119
dextran, 119
diabetics, 51
dialysis, 91
diapedesis, 41, 148
differentiation, 6
diffusion, 10, 51, 148
diphosphoglycerate (2,3-DPG), 34, 148
disease transmission, 79, 80, 97-102
disseminated intravascular coagulation
    (DIC), 27, 72-74, 148
    causes, 72
    clot lysis, 72
    coagulation factor consumption, 72
    diagnosis, 74
    management, 74
    platelet consumption and, 76-77
    signs and symptoms, 73
donation, blood, 79-81, 149
    donor diseases, 79-80, 97-102

edema, 12, 57, 104
electrolytes, 149

in plasma, 48, 50
endothelial cells and growth factors, 6
endothelial damage, 53, 72
endothelium, 8, 149
enzyme-linked immunosorbent assay
  (ELISA), 100, 149
enzyme (protein) cascade. *See* coagulation
  cascade
eosinophils, 42, 43, 149
Epstein-Barr (EBV), 97
erythrocytes, 1, 31-34, 149. *See also* red blood
  cells
erythrocytosis, 35
erythropoietin (EPO) growth factor, 6, 112,
  149
erythropoietin and erythropoiesis, 37, 112,
  149
exchange transfusion, 29
extramedullary hematopoeisis, 5, 149
extravascular, 8, 149
extrinsic pathway of coagulation, 59, 64-67

febrile transfusion reaction, 95
fetus and Rh antigen, 28-29
fibrin, 61-67, 149
  clot, 53, 55, 57, 61
  degradation products (FDPs), 68
  glue, 110, 149
  split products (FSPs), 68, 73
  stabilization, 61
fibrinogen (factor I), 51, 73, 149
fibrinolysis, 149
fibroblasts, 5, 6
filtration, 10, 149
  of blood, 85-86
fluids. *See* lymphatic system; vascular system
fluid balance, 50
Flood and Drug Administration (FDA), 83,
  97
formed elements, 1, 37, 51, 85
forward (cell) typing, 84
fresh frozen plasma (FFP), 62, 73, 149
  and component therapy, 109, 110, 114

G-CSF and GM-CSF, 112-113
gamma globulin, 111, 149-150
globin, 150
globulin, 150
glucose in plasma, 50
gonococcus, 19

genetic defects in vascular wall, 71
graft-versus-host disease (GVHD), 45, 150
granulocytes, 17, 107, 150
  and component therapy, 114
  types of, 42
granulocyte colony-stimulating factor (G-
  CSF), 6, 112-113
granulocyte-macrophage colony-stimulating
  factor (GM-CSF), 6, 112-113
growth factors, 6, 104, 111-113

H+, 150
heart, 12-15. *See also* cardiopulmonary
  system; circulatory system
  coronary thrombosis, 58
  hepatitis, 81, 97-99, 150-151
  valves, 67
hemapheresis, 105
hematocrit (Hct), 37, 80, 150
hematology, 1, 150
hematopoiesis, 2, 5, 150
hematopoietic (red) marrow, 3, 5
heme, 31
hemodilution, 122, 150
hemoglobin (Hgb), 31-34, 37, 80, 90, 150
  diphosphoglycerate (2,3-DPG), 34
  normal concentrations, 33
  oxygen, affinity for 33-34
  plasma-free, 38, 90, 154
hemolysis, 21-22, 38, 84-85, 90, 91, 150
hemolytic disease of the newborn (HDN),
  29, 150
hemolytic transfusion reaction, 25, 27, 90-94
hemophilia, 1, 64, 71, 79, 83, 150
hemorrhagic disorders, 71, 150
hemostasis, 53, 55-59, 61, 150
  ADP release, 57-58
  platelet function in coagulation, 56, 57-58
  vascular spasm, 55, 57
heparin, 44, 123, 150
hepatitis, 150-151
  blood donors, 80, 97, 98
  hepatitis B (HVB), 81, 98-99
  hepatitis B immune globulin (HBIG), 99,
    151
  hepatitis B vaccine, 98-99, 151
  hepatitis C, 81, 97, 98
  testing for, 81, 97
  transfusion and, 98-99

viruses in *Hepadnaviridae* family, 98
hetastarch, 119
histamine, 19, 44, 151
HIV. See human immunodeficiency virus
(HIV)
HLA. See human leukocyte antigens (HLA)
host-versus-graft disease, 45, 151
HTLV-I/II (human T cell lymphotropic
virus), 81, 97, 102
human immunodeficiency virus (HIV), 151
acquired immune deficiency syndrome
(AIDS) and, 99-102
blood testing, 80-81, 97, 99-100
enzyme-linked immunoassay (ELISA)
blood test, 100
Western blot blood test, 100
and transfusions, 80, 81, 97, 99-100
human leukocyte antigens (HLA/MHC), 85,
105, 107, 151
human T cell lymphotropic virus (HTLV-I/
II), 81, 97, 102
humoral immunity, 46
humoral immune response, 19-20, 151
hydrostatic pressure, 151
hypervolemia, 151
hypogammaglobulinemia, 111, 151
hypotension, 27
hypothermia, 151
hypovolemia, 111, 151
hypoxia, 37, 151
hemolytic disease of newborn (HDN), 29

IgA antibody, 19
IgD antibody, 18
IgE antibody, 18-29
IgG antibody, 19, 23
IgM antibody, 18, 23
immune response, 17-21, 76, 152
HIV/AIDS and, 101-102
hemolysis and, 38
white blood cells and, 42, 45
immune serum globulin, 111, 115
immune system, 17-23, 152
antibodies, classes of, 18-19
antigens, 17-18
complement system, 21-23
function of, 17
humoral and cell-mediated responses, 19-
21, 46, 148, 151
phagocytosis, 20-21, 41

Rh antigen, 27-29
and saccharide-coated organisms, 19
suppression, 45
white blood cells, function in, 5, 41-46
immunoglobulins, 18, 152. See also antibodies, immune system
in vitro coagulation experiments, 64
in vivo coagulation experiments, 64
infection. See also immune response; immune
system
and cell-mediated responses, 19-21
increased white blood cell production, 3
inferior vena cava, 13, 14, 152
insulin, 51
interstitial
fluid, 48
space, 8, 12, 48, 152
intraoperative blood salvage, 123-125
intramedullary hematopoeisis, 5
intravascular, 8, 152
intravenous. See also transfusion
intrinsic pathway of coagulation, 59, 64-67
ITP (idiopathic thrombocytopenia), 109
I.V. See also transfusion solution, 87

kidneys
kidney cells and growth factors, 6, 112
role in increasing red blood cells, 36, 37
transfusion reactions, 91
Kupffer's cells, 68

labile factors, 83
lactated Ringer's, 119
Landsteiner, Karl, 25
left atrium (LA), 14
left ventricle (LV), 14
leukemia, 97, 152
leukocytes, 1, 41, 152. See also white blood
cells
depletion, 85, 107
leukocyte-adsorption filters, 85
leukocyte-depletion filters, 85
leukocyte-poor red blood cells, 107, 152
liver
and clotting factors, 62, 64
diseases and blood testing, 76, 97-99
failure and fibrin split products (FSPs), 68
fetal blood cell development, 3
Kuppfer's cells, 68, 73
white blood cells in, 44

lungs, 14-15, 50. *See also* circulatory system
  white blood cells in, 43, 44
lymph, 12, 152
lymph nodes, 10-12, 46, 152
lymphadenopathy, 101, 152
lymphatic channels, 10
lymphatic system, 10-12, 44, 152
lymphocytes, 45, 152
  differentiation of, 42, 45
  function in immune response, 17, 45-46
  growth factors, 6
  organ rejection and, 45
  types, 42, 46
lymphoma, 97
lysis
  of antigen, 19, 22, 45
  of clot, 55, 68
lysosomes, 41, 44

macrophages, 42, 44, 152. *See also* monocytes
  function in immune response, 17, 20, 44
  growth factors, 6
major histocompatibility/human leukocyte
  antigen (MHL/HLA), 85
malaria, 80, 97, 152
mannitol, 83
Marfan's syndrome, 71
megakaryocyte, 53, 153
membrane attack complex (MAC), 23
meningococcus, 19
MHL/HLA (major histocompatibility/human
  leukocyte antigen), 85. *See also* human
  leukocyte antigen
microaggregate blood filters, 85
microorganisms and immune system, 17-18
mitochondria, 33
mitral valve, 14
monocytes, 42, 44, 153. *See also* macrophages
monomers, 67
mononuclear phagocytic system (Kupffer's
  cells), 68, 153
mucus, 153
mucous membranes, antibody protection of,
  19

neutrophils, 20, 42, 43, 153
newborns
  hemolytic disease of the newborn (HDN),
  29
  and hepatitis, 98

nonwash device, 123, 125, 153
normal saline, 87, 118-119, 122
normovolemia, 104
normovolemic anemia, 122
nucleus, 31, 153
numbers (count)
  CD4+T in AIDS, 100
  platelets, 53, 76-77
  red blood cells, 35
  white blood cells, 42

O blood group, 25-27, 90, 153
oncotic pressure, 48
opportunistic infection, 101, 153
opsonin, 18
opsonization, 18, 22, 43, 153
organ rejection, 45, 153
osmosis, 153
osmotic pressure, 12, 48
oxygen, 153
  and blood cell production, 2-3
  and red blood cells, 5, 21, 31-34
oxygenation
  of blood, 14, 31-34, 153
  of tissues, 33-34, 38

packed red cells, 25, 79, 82, 85, 104, 106-107,
  114, 153
parasite, 43, 153
passive immunity, 111, 153-154
PCO_2 (partial pressure of carbon dioxide), 34
perfuse/perfusion, 33-34, 154
peripheral circulation, 13
pH, 34, 48, 50, 154
phagocyte, 18, 41, 43, 44, 154
phagocytosis, 20-21, 154
  in humoral and cell-mediated responses, 20-
  21
  process, 20, 41, 43, 44
phosphate, 81-82
phospholipids, 154
  binding via calcium bridge, 62, 64
  function in coagulation, 57
  platelets and DIC, 72
plasma, 1-2, 48-51, 90, 154
  albumin and plasma protein fraction (PPF),
  110-111, 115
  antibodies in, 18, 25, 99
  component therapy, 104, 109-111

composition of, 48-51
function of, 49
fresh frozen (FFP), 62, 73, 109, 110, 149
proteins, 12, 21, 48
removal from donated blood, 82
and serum, 51
plasma cell, 18, 20, 46, 154
plasma-free hemoglobin, 38, 90, 125, 154
plasma protein fraction (PPF), 110-111, 115
plasmapheresis, 105, 106
plasmin and plasminogen, 68, 154
platelet count test, 76
platelet factor 3, 58
platelet membrane phospholipipd, 62, 64
    binding via calcium bridge, 62
    extrinsic pathway, 64-67
    intrinsic pathway, 63-66
platelet plug. *See* platelets
plateletpheresis, 105
platelets (thrombocytes), 1, 5, 53, 154
    aggregation, 57, 58, 72
    apheresis, 108
    and component therapy, 104, 108-109,
    114
    function in coagulation, 57
    increased production after blood loss, 3
    lifespan, 53
    and phospholipids, 57-59
    plug, 5, 53, 55, 57, 58
    quantity and quality, 76-77
    size and count, 53, 76-77
    storage, 109
    and white cells, 85
    transfusions, 74, 108-109
pluripotential stem cell, 6
pneumococcus, 19
polycythemia, 35, 154
pooled platelets, 154
pore size, blood filter, 85, 154
postoperative wound drainage, 125
potassium in plasma, 50
predonation of blood, 121, 154
pregnancy and Rh antigen, 27-29
preservatives, 81-82
prostacyclin (PGI$_2$), 58
prostaglandins, 58
protein in plasma, 12, 21, 48
protein receptor (binding site), 6
pulmonary artery, 14
pulmonary valve, 14

pulmonary veins, 15

reagents, 84
receptor, 6, 46
recombinant growth factors, 105, 111-113
recombinant technology, 112
red blood cells, 1, 3, 5, 31-38
    count, health problems due to, 35, 57
    diphosphoglycurate (2,3-DPG), 34
    enucleated, 31
    erythopoietin, 37
    formation, 31
    function of hemoglobin, 31-34
    grouping and cross matching, 84-85
    hematocrit, 37
    heme molecule in, 31
    lifespan, 31
    membrane, 25, 38
    production, 3
    red cell hemolysis, 38
    shape and number of, 35, 57
    viability of, and preservatives, 81
Red Cross, 83
red marrow, 3, 5, 154
rejection, organ, 45, 153
renal failure, 91, 155
renal tubular necrosis, 91
neticulocndothelial cells (Kupffer's cells), 68,
    153 *See also* mononuclear phagocytic system
reticuloendothelial system (RES), 68, 155
retroviruses, 155
reverse (serum) typing, 84
Rh antigen, 27-29, 155
    determination, 85
    transfusion reaction, 27-29, 90
Rh immune globulin, 29, 108
right atrium (RA), 13-14
right lymphatic duct, 12, 155
right ventricle (RV), 14

self-renewal, 6
sepsis, 38, 95
septicemia, 155
serine proteases, 61, 155
serology blood tests, 51
seronegative blood, 97
seropositive blood, 97
serum, 51, 84, 85, 155
shunting, 57
single-donor apheresis, 105, 155

sinusoids, 44
sodium in plasma, 50
solutes in plasma, 48
spleen
 function of, 38
 and platelets, 53
 fetal blood cell production in, 3
 white blood cells in, 44
stable factors, 83
stem (progenitor) cells, 155
 cellular differentiation, 6
 differentiated and undifferentiated, 6
 production in bone marrow, 2-3, 5-6, 37
stored blood. *See* banked (stored) blood
stress, red cell membrane, 38
stroke prevention, 58, 68
stroma
 bone, 3
 hemolysis, 38
superior vena cava, 13, 14, 155
surgery
 and methods of autologous blood recovery,
 121, 125
 and pathways of coagulation, 64
 wash and nonwash devices, 123-125
syphilis, 81, 97
synthetic volume expanders, 118-119

T cells, 19, 42, 44, 46, 155
 and cell-mediated responses, 19-20, 46
 CD4+, 101-102
 CD8+, 148
target cell. *See* phagocytosis
testing donated blood, 81, 97-99
therapeutic apheresis, 106
thoracic duct, 12, 155
thrombin, 67, 155
thrombocytes, 53, 155. *See also* platelets
 (thrombocytes)
thrombocytosis and thrombocytopenia, 53,
 76-77, 108, 155
thromboplastin, 59, 62, 65, 67, 155-156
thrombotic disorder, 71, 156
Thromboxane A$_2$, 58
thymus, 3, 46
tissue membrane phospholipid (tissue
 thromboplastin), 62, 65, 67
 binding via calcium bridge, 62
tissue perfusion (oxygenation), 33-34, 82, 154
tissue plasminogen activator (TPA), 68, 156

titer, 99, 100
total blood volume, 1, 81
transfusion, 79-87
 additive systems, 82-83
 anticoagulants, 79, 81-82
 apheresis, 105-106
 autologous blood recovery methods, 79,
 121-125
 autotransfusion, 121
 blood administration, 86-87
 blood donation for, 79-81. *See also* banked
 (stored) blood
 blood filtering, 85-86
 blood grouping and cross matching, 84-85
 blood testing, 81, 97, 100
 citrate anticoagulants/preservatives (CPD,
 CP2D, CPDA-1), 81-82, 123, 107
 coagulation factors and, 61-67
 compatibility, 25-27, 79, 84-84
 component therapy and, 104-113
 disease transmission, 79, 97-102
 exchange to prevent hemolytic disease of
 the newborn (HDN), 29
 and HIV infection (AIDS virus), 80, 81, 97,
 99-102
 platelet, 108-109
 therapy, 79
transfusion reactions, 25, 27, 70, 86-95, 156
 signs and symptoms (tables), 92-95
tricuspid valve, 14
tubing set for blood administration, 86-87

universal donor/recipient, 27
undifferentiated cells, 6

vaccine, 156
 hepatitis B vaccine, 98-99
vascular integrity, 71, 72, 156
vascular permeability, 22
vascular space, 8, 48, 156. *See also* vascular
 system
vascular spasm, 55, 57
vascular system, 3, 8-12, 13-15, 156
 cardiopulmonary system, 14-15
 disorders, 71
 fluid (blood) volume, 1-2, 12, 48, 118, 121
 peripheral circulation, 13
 plasma in, 48
 origin, 3
vasculature, 156

vasculitis, 156
veins, 8, 13, 57, 81
vena cavae, superior and inferior, 13, 14
venule end, 10, 12
venules, 13
viremia, 156
virus, 20, 156. *See also* acquired immune
    deficiency syndrome; hepatitis, T lympho-
    cyte tropic virus
    intracellular attack, 20
vitamin K, 67, 156
    deficiency, 72
volume expanders, 118-119
von Willebrand's disease, 76

warfarin, 67, 156
wash and nonwash devices, 123-125, 153, 156
Western blot test, 100, 156
white blood cells, 1, 5, 41-46
    basophils, 44
    and component therapy, 107-108
    eosinophils, 43
    filters, 85-86
    function in immune system, 5, 17, 19-21, 41
    lymphocytes, 45
    monocytes/macrophages, 44
    neutrophils, 43
    number, 42
    production, 3
    properties, 41
    T cell and B cells, 46
    types, 42
whole blood, 2, 81, 82, 83, 104-105, 114, 156-
    157
wound drainage, 125

yellow marrow, 3, 5, 157
yolk sac, 3